Praise for

Praise for
The Emotional Eating, Chronic Dieting, Binge Eating, and Body Image Workbook

"I am so grateful to Matz, Pershing, and Harrison for joining forces on this phenomenal workbook. I hear every day from folks in desperate need of this very resource, and these authors have the expertise, experience, and compassion to do this work justice."

—**Virginia Sole-Smith,** *New York Times* bestselling author of *Fat Talk*

"For much of my life, I believed the lie that the size of my body was something to be 'fixed.' The endless pursuit of weight loss through my teenage years into my twenties left me with poor health, debilitating body shame, a suicide attempt, and a years-long eating disorder. In my own journey to fat liberation and health at every size, all three of these authors have published texts and resources respectively that changed my life and granted me a freedom I did not know was possible, so it should come as no surprise that powerhouse trio Judith Matz, Amy Pershing, and Christy Harrison have created a groundbreaking resource that addresses so many aspects of the harm that weight loss fixation has done on our culture. With a wealth of evidence-based information, practical approaches to countering body shame, and disordered eating, and thoughtful space for individuals and clinicians to be curious about their own experiences, it's doubly impressive that the book's language is so accessible. I cannot wait to bring this text to my workshops!"

—**Mary Lambert,** Grammy-nominated singer/songwriter and body positive activist

"*The Emotional Eating, Chronic Dieting, Binge Eating, and Body Image Workbook* is a comprehensive resource for learning how diet culture impacts you and practicing how to navigate it all with compassion instead of quick fixes that don't last. This is the kind of workbook that serves as foundational knowledge to equip you throughout your life and as a go-to resource for immediate advice or strategies at the moment you need them."

—**Lexie Kite, PhD,** co-author of *More Than a Body: Your Body Is an Instrument, Not an Ornament*

"Matz, Pershing, and Harrison have constructed a workbook that lays an important foundation for further work on recovery from eating disorders, disordered eating, and chronic dieting. The combined expertise of the authors delivers the perfect balance of knowledge needed for those struggling with the relationship to their bodies in a culture that assigns value based on the shape and size of individuals."

—**Chevese Turner,** founder and CEO of Body Equity Alliance, founder and former CEO of Binge Eating Disorder Association, and co-author of *Binge Eating Disorder: The Journey to Recovery and Beyond*

"Superstar clinicians and authors Matz, Pershing, and Harrison have gifted us with this practical, useful, and healing workbook. It reveals with compassion the dangers and damage of diet culture and weight stigma, then offers instead the most scientifically and psychologically sound best practices. This is a brilliant resource for individuals looking for the truest pathway toward a joyful and sustainable relationship with eating as well as being an invaluable tool for clinicians to use with clients."

—**Jennifer L. Gaudiani, MD, CEDS-S, FAED,** founder and medical director of the Gaudiani Clinic and author of *Sick Enough: A Guide to the Medical Complications of Eating Disorders*

"Finally, a workbook specifically for the most common eating issues plaguing us—emotional eating, chronic dieting, and bingeing. With just enough scientific background to understand the origins of our disordered eating, this resource companions us through the process of slowing down and stretching out compressed moments so that we can really feel our bodily sensations and emotions and see our thoughts and actions in real time. When we see ourselves clearly and honestly, we can course-correct! By doing the thoughtful contemplations and personalized intention-setting, you will start to see yourself healing a lifetime of harmful thought patterns and behaviors in a sustainable way!"

—**Jenna Hollenstein, MS, RD,** author of *Eat to Love: A Mindful Guide to Transforming Your Relationship with Food, Body, and Life* and *Intuitive Eating for Life: How Mindfulness Can Deepen and Sustain Your Intuitive Eating Practice*

"If you struggle with emotional eating, chronic dieting, binge eating, or a difficult relationship with food—this workbook is for you! And if you are a professional working with these issues, this book is for you too! Judith Matz, Amy Pershing, and Christy Harrison are renowned experts in the field of eating disorders; they use their collective wisdom to clearly explain the cultural forces that contribute to disordered eating and teach practical tools and strategies to help you improve your relationship with food. The book is filled with exercises and prompts to help you engage deeply in the work. This is a valuable resource I'll be recommending to clients and clinicians alike!"

—**Alexis Consason, PsyD, CEDS-C,** clinical psychologist and author of *The Diet-Free Revolution: 10 Steps to Free Yourself from the Diet Cycle with Mindful Eating and Radical Self-Acceptance*

"This workbook addresses the vicious cycle of negative self-perception, restrictive eating, emotional eating, chronic dieting, and bingeing caused by an obsession with unrealistic body ideals and dieting culture. Through insightful guidance and practical exercises, readers embark on a transformative journey to break free from damaging effects of dieting and forge a compassionate relationship with food and body. Clinicians will also find value from insightful reflections providing strategies for supporting clients' healing journey."

—**Hilary Kinavey, MS, LPC,** co-author of *Reclaiming Body Trust: A Path to Healing and Liberation*

"The Emotional Eating, Chronic Dieting, Binge Eating, and Body Image Workbook will benefit those wanting to move away from chronic dieting to a more positive relationship with food and their body as well as professionals who are supporting clients in that work. We are all impacted by messages that tell us our body isn't acceptable and that we need to be constantly trying to 'fix' it. This workbook will support readers in recognizing how these messages have interfered with them developing a compassionate relationship with food and their body. Readers will learn from three leaders in their field and have the opportunity to reflect on what they read with thought-provoking and insightful journal prompts and questions. This workbook is also a great tool for professionals who work with clients around these topics. Each chapter has a section specifically for professionals that will be helpful in guiding work with clients. I highly recommend this workbook to anyone who is tired of chronic dieting, body hatred, or negative body image and would like to find a different way forward."

—**Rachel Millner, PsyD, CEDS-S,** licensed psychologist, certified eating
disorder specialist and supervisor, and certified Body Trust® provider

"The Emotional Eating, Chronic Dieting, Binge Eating, and Body Image Workbook is more than a workbook; it's a supportive companion on the path to rediscovering joy and balance in one's relationship with food and self. It will empower you to redefine health on your terms, embracing a life free from judgment and filled with self-compassion. In addition to helping individuals, clinicians will find immense value in this workbook as it provides insightful reflections at the end of each chapter, enriching the professional toolkit with practical strategies for supporting clients on their journey to healing."

—**Aaron Flores, RDN,** certified Body Trust® provider

"Judith, Amy, and Christy are renowned authors and experienced clinicians who've put together a fantastic resource for people looking to explore internalized narratives around food and their bodies and ultimately find peace."

—**Dana Sturtevant MS, RD,** co-author of *Reclaiming Body Trust: A Path to Healing and Liberation*

"From three recognized experts, *The Emotional Eating, Chronic Dieting, Binge Eating, and Body Image Workbook* is a practical, accessible guide to breaking free of the diet cycle. It provides a great overview of the non-diet landscape and thought-provoking writing reflections to help readers consider and apply these concepts in their own lives. A huge bonus: the Clinician's Corner at end of each chapter helps health professionals explore how diet culture affects them personally and professionally."

—**Michelle May,** author of the *Eat What You Love, Love What You Eat* book series
and founder of Am I Hungry? Mindful Eating Programs and Training

"This workbook is a gentle and wise accompaniment for those who want to learn to relate to food and their bodies with more respect and care. The authors skillfully and compassionately guide us through thoughtful reflections and practical suggestions, orienting us towards a relationship with our bodies that holds the possibility of more freedom."

—**Carmen Cool, MA, LPC, CHT,** psychotherapist

"An excellent workbook by three distinguished experts in the field. A resource like this that is both trauma-informed and weight-inclusive is a true gift to the world and will help countless people repair and improve their relationships with food and their bodies."

—**Ragen Chastain,** health coach and author of the Weight and Healthcare newsletter on Substack

The Emotional Eating, Chronic Dieting, Binge Eating & Body Image Workbook

A Trauma-Informed, Weight-Inclusive Approach to Make Peace with Food & Reduce Body Shame

Judith Matz, LCSW, ACSW • Amy Pershing, LMSW, ACSW, CCTP-II
Christy Harrison, MPH, RD, CEDS

Published by
PESI Publishing, Inc.
3839 White Ave
Eau Claire, WI 54703

Cover and interior design by Amy Rubenzer
Editing by Jenessa Jackson, PhD

ISBN 9781683737223 (print)
ISBN 9781683737230 (ePUB)
ISBN 9781683737247 (ePDF)

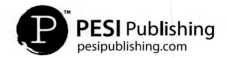

PESI Publishing
pesipublishing.com

Table of Contents

Introduction

Do you find yourself upset when you eat foods that you believe are "bad" for you? Do you consider yourself to be an "emotional eater"? Does eating ever feel out of control for you? Have you tried multiple diets, only to regain the weight? These are common experiences for millions of people, and often the recommended solution is to try a new diet or wellness plan. But what if these plans and programs are actually part of the problem? As clinicians, we've witnessed firsthand the harm that results when people are told, "Just try harder," "It's a matter of willpower," or even "Healing your emotional issues will result in weight loss."

Dieting to lose weight can take up a lot of your time, energy, and money. It can leave you feeling on top of the world when you feel in control of your food choices and like a failure when you eat the very foods you've been trying to avoid. But what if that "failure" isn't your fault? The fact is that while just about all diets work in the short run, upward of 95 percent of people will regain the weight over time, with one-third to two-thirds ending up above their pre-diet weight. If you know someone who has lost weight and kept it off permanently, they are a unicorn!

We also understand that because of societal messages that value thinness as a sign of worthiness, there's a good chance you feel shame about your body or your relationship with food. You may have tried to change your body size through the pursuit of weight loss over a period of months, years, or even decades. You may rely on food to get you through times of distress. You may believe that once you achieve the "correct" body size, everything in your life will get better.

We invite you to take a moment to reflect on which of the following statements describe your situation:

- I can maintain a diet for a period of time but then find myself eating the very foods I tried to avoid.

- I turn to food when I experience emotional distress.

- I need to lose weight to be happy and successful in life.

- My eating feels out of control at times.

- I am worried about my physical health because of my eating or my body size.

If you agreed with one or more of these statements, this workbook is for you! We wrote this book to provide you with a path to freedom from chronic dieting, emotional and binge eating, and body shame. The path we offer is compassionate, trauma-informed, and research-based. In these pages, you'll find a wealth of information, strategies, and stories to help you heal your relationship with food and feel more at home in your body. With the tools inside, you'll learn to:

- Eat in a way that nourishes your body and gives you pleasure, without the feelings of anxiety, guilt, and deprivation that usually accompany weight loss and so-called wellness plans

- Trust your body to know what it needs to feel comfortable and satiated

- Understand the role that food plays in your life and learn new ways to connect with yourself and meet your needs

- Take care of your body in ways that support physical and emotional well-being, without the shame of diet failure

- End the preoccupation with food and weight so you free up your mental energy

This path takes patience, compassion, and curiosity, but we've heard from the thousands of clients we've worked with over the decades that it's well worth the journey. We're so glad you're here.

What to Expect from This Book

This workbook is divided into three main sections: (1) understanding the problem, (2) learning new strategies, and (3) finding solutions. Section 1 explores the backdrop of diet culture, describes how you've gotten stuck in the diet cycle, and explains why diet failure isn't your fault.

Section 2 offers a wealth of information and activities to support you in healing your relationship with food and your body. You'll learn how to reconnect with your body so that food becomes a source of nourishment and pleasure instead of creating anxiety and discomfort. You'll also explore how to respond to emotional eating and binge eating disorder (BED) with curiosity and compassion rather than blame and shame so that you can find ways to effectively heal your relationship with food. With an understanding of how diet culture impacts your body image, you'll learn strategies to reduce body shame and feel more at home in your body.

Finally, section 3 addresses topics such as health and weight stigma to help you build the skills and resilience that lead to greater physical and emotional well-being. Ultimately, our hope is that this workbook allows you to live more fully in the world and helps to create a more weight-inclusive culture.

Although we primarily wrote this workbook to help individuals working on their own to make peace with food and their bodies, it also can be used by clinicians, who may recommend it as a supplementary resource for clients or as an important tool to use within individual or group sessions.

If you are using this book to support your own healing journey, we recommend moving at your own pace as you make your way through the information, strategies, and exercises offered throughout. If you feel overwhelmed by what you're learning, you can slow down. If the order of chapters isn't a good match for your process, skip to where you need to be (with the caveat that chapter 8, which offers information about gentle nutrition, is best explored after you've digested the preceding chapters). We believe that you know what's best for you. At the same time, we also want to gently acknowledge that rejecting the diet mindset and shifting to the approaches offered in this book can feel relieving *and* scary at the same time. If you get stuck along the way, remember to check in with yourself and see what would support you in continuing with your journey to heal your relationship with food and your body.

If you are a professional working with clients, we have a special section at the end of each chapter called *Clinician's Corner* where we offer information, advice, or wisdom related to the content you've just read. We understand that you've grown up in the same diet culture as your clients, and you may be struggling with the same issues we explore throughout this workbook. You may decide to use the tools inside to address your own eating and body concerns before you start to share new ideas with your clients.

Even if you don't feel ready to teach these concepts, as you become aware of how diet culture frequently results in physical and emotional harm, you can make sure that you don't—even inadvertently—contribute to the shame your clients experience around food and body size. We, too, believed in diets early in our own careers and used to prescribe weight loss plans to our clients. We each made a shift as we witnessed diet failure with our clients, prompting us to take a deeper look at the research. As you get more comfortable with an anti-diet approach, you'll find that the information, strategies, and exercises in these pages can be tailored to meet your clients' needs. And, of course, if you're already familiar with the approach offered in this workbook, we hope that this resource will become a valuable complement to the work you're already doing.

We invite you to approach our workbook with openness and curiosity. Diet culture may have taught you that your worthiness is based on your body shape and size, but that's simply not true. These messages and beliefs about food and weight are all around us, but they can be explored and unlearned so that you can make peace with food and reduce body shame. It is our deepest hope that these pages will offer you the guidance you need to begin (or continue) your journey of healing your relationship with food and your body or to support others on this life-changing path.

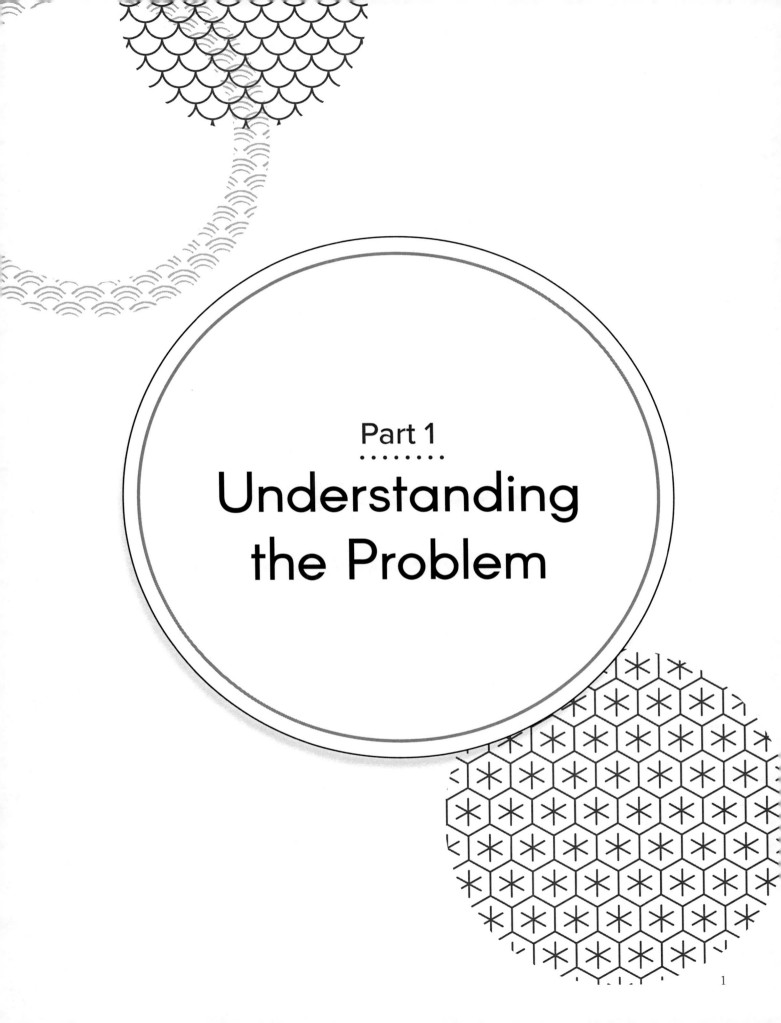

Part 1

Understanding the Problem

CHAPTER 1

The Problem with Diet Culture

Diet culture encompasses the messages, attitudes, and values related to body size and eating. It awards status to thinner people and assumes that eating in a certain way will result in the "correct" body size and good health for everyone who has the dedication to stick to it. Diet culture treats eating the "right" foods as a moral issue, leading to culturally induced fat shaming, weight stigma, and body shame. Diet culture affects all of us—as well as our families, friends, colleagues, and even health care providers.

It is virtually impossible to grow up in our culture and *not* take in these messages. No matter your age, race, ethnicity, gender, ability, or other identities, we are all living in diet culture. Sadly, this prompts many of us to disconnect from our bodies in an effort to achieve a cultural ideal. While weight loss is often viewed as a matter of willpower, the reality is that diets are almost always guaranteed to fail due to strong physiological and psychological forces that are part of being human. We'll get to those details later in the workbook, but for now we want you to know that when you can't maintain your diet, *it isn't your fault*. It's not fair when you're blamed—even shamed—for weight regain. Your diet has actually set you up for that result.

What Is *Your* Story?

When it comes to food, weight, and body image, everyone has a story. We'd like to start by sharing our own stories.

Judith's Story: The Deprivation of Diets

• • •

When I was in high school, all the girls I knew were dieting. I was thin, but I became terrified of gaining weight, so I started to diet for the first time. I stopped eating anything that I thought was "fattening" and instead started skipping meals and eating foods like plain yogurt, which I hated. As I continued to diet, I also started to binge for the first time. An entire Sarah Lee banana cake. A can of pink frosting. This was upsetting, so I tried to diet harder.

I continued to diet all through my college and graduate school years, and the pattern of bingeing also continued. My body changed such that I was described as "Rubenesque" by a male friend who felt free to comment.

In my early twenties, I spent a summer in Boston to experience living in a new city before returning to my "real" life in the Chicago area. I got a job as a waitress at a well-known seafood restaurant where food was both plentiful and delicious. I discovered a shop that had ice cream with Oreo cookie mix-ins—something that was brand new at the time. I was living in a tiny studio apartment with no mirror or scale, and I had the thought: *I'm so sick of dieting—I'm going to take the summer off from that too.*

To my surprise, by the end of the summer my bingeing had stopped! I had an "aha" moment as I understood that my food restrictions had set me up to binge, and I made this promise to myself: If I ever had the thought that I shouldn't eat something because it was too high in calories, I would eat it to prove to myself that I could. No more deprivation because of my fear of fat.

I was fortunate to have grown up in a family where my parents didn't go on diets or restrict what I ate, and we could afford a wide variety of foods. I wasn't an "emotional eater," so I was returning to the way I ate growing up. I never experienced stigma because of my body size, but I did feel the pressure to diet, and I'm so grateful I made the connection between the deprivation of diets and bingeing early in my life. Since then, it's become my life's work to help others understand that they haven't failed their diet; their diet has failed them.

Amy's Story: Finding Body Compassion

• • •

I was considered "chubby" as a kid, and so was my mom. She put me on my first diet when I was 9 years old. Her goal was for me to avoid the body shame she felt growing up, and the best way she knew to do that was to help me lose weight. Thus began decades of working to make my body conform to a shape and size I was told it should be. My body never maintained the weight I lost without severe restriction, and I simply saw this as a sign to try harder.

In those many years of dieting, I learned that hunger was virtuous, that fullness meant I had failed, and that regardless of the amount of weight I lost, I could never really be thin enough. As a result, and because of other difficult experiences in my life, I developed binge eating disorder in my teens. I did not know I had an eating disorder at the time; I just thought I had no self-control. Little did I know that, along with other traumatic experiences, my dieting and body shame were direct causes of my binge eating. It took many years for me to realize that I would need to build trust and compassion for my body before I could truly heal.

With a lot of hard work in therapy and support from others along the way, I recovered from my eating disorder many years ago. A critical part of the journey was learning that my body actually knows how to feel satisfied by food and movement and that it will tell me what it needs if I listen closely. I discovered that my body will always know itself better than any diet. Regardless of my shape, weight, or current health concerns, I've come to have immense compassion and gratitude for the body I have. I've learned, too, that it is not my body's job to be acceptable to others or meet some external standard; my body is first and foremost my home, deserving of the very best care I can offer. I hope this workbook will help you find a more peaceful and gentle relationship with food and your own body too. Here's to your journey!

Christy's Story: Disordered Eating and the Search for Wellness

• • •

I was lucky to grow up as an intuitive eater. My family always had enough to eat, and I've always been relatively thin, so no one interfered with my relationship with food by telling me I needed to lose weight. I still absorbed many of the weight-stigmatizing messages of the diet culture around me, including the idea that my large appetite was only a good thing because I was thin. I also had body insecurities that popped up after I went through puberty and started reading teen magazines. But I never dieted or worried about my weight.

All of that changed at age 20, when I went on a yearlong study-abroad program to Paris. Early on, I gained a little bit of weight, thanks to a new birth control pill, and suddenly I became painfully aware of all the diet culture messages I'd unconsciously absorbed throughout my life. I struggled to eat less, to control the appetite that now felt like a liability. By the middle of my second semester in that program, I was engaging in some disordered eating and exercise behaviors. When I returned home, in the summer of 2002, I started my first official diet.

Within a few months, I started bingeing almost every night, then restricting and exercising even harder the next day to try to compensate—behaviors that I only much later realized amounted to a diagnosable eating disorder, though I unfortunately never got help at the time. Instead, I saw myself as out of control, an emotional eater who just needed to "get my act together," rather than someone responding to the deep, desperate hunger that food deprivation had caused.

I soon started having health problems—missed periods, abdominal pain, dry skin, fatigue, brain fog—and started going from doctor to doctor to figure out what was going on. I couldn't see that my restrictive eating was at the root of most of my issues, and I searched in vain for food sensitivities or other diagnoses to explain them, dabbling in alternative and functional medicine approaches that only led me further into disordered eating. Along the way, I did manage to find some good doctors who diagnosed me with a number of real, chronic conditions, including Hashimoto's thyroiditis (an autoimmune disease that causes low thyroid levels), irritable bowel syndrome, gastroesophageal reflux disease, and later several more autoimmune, hormonal, and digestive disorders. But none of those conditions entirely explained the symptoms I was experiencing, which left me frustrated and vulnerable to dubious approaches that blamed food for all my ills.

Meanwhile, I was working as a journalist covering food, nutrition, and health, trying to figure out and report on the "healthiest" ways to eat. It wasn't until six years into my career that I finally started to explore my own disordered relationship with food in therapy. With the support of a wonderful therapist, alongside my own journalistic research on emotional eating, I slowly began treating myself with more compassion and eased up on my food restrictions. As I did, I started to experience greater peace and ease with food and saw a slow but steady reduction in my symptoms. I began to reconnect with the intuitive eating I'd known for the first two decades of my life.

Healing from disordered eating certainly wasn't a straight line (I don't think it is for anyone), but today my relationship with food is better than ever, and I'm committed to helping others recover from the issues I struggled with. I hope this workbook helps you on your own path toward discovery, reflection, and healing.

Now that you know our stories, what is *your* story? Take some time to reflect on what you've experienced and how you want to tell it. We've given you some space here to write your story. If you need more room, grab some sheets of paper. Or perhaps you'd prefer to type on your computer or write in a journal. Choose what works best for you.

Notice how you feel as you write your story.

_____

_____

_____

_____

_____

_____

_____

_____

_____

_____

_____

_____

Now that you're done, add a title that captures what you've written.

Is there anyone you want to share your story with at this time?

Consider putting your story away for a week or two and then coming back to it. How do you feel when you read it again?

Your story matters.

The Language of Diet Culture

Problems with food can show up in all sorts of ways. Let's look at some ways people struggle in their relationship with food:

- The diet mindset
- Rebound eating
- Chronic dieting
- Emotional eating

- Binge eating disorder
- Disordered eating
- Orthorexia

The Diet Mindset

Diet culture's outlook on food and weight is so prevalent that you may not realize you're seeing the world through its lens. This way of thinking is referred to as the *diet mindset*. Here are some common statements that come from the diet mindset:

- "I'm being 'good' today," referring to what you eat.
- "Today is a cheat day."
- "I need to lose weight for the wedding/for my health/to fit back into my jeans."
- "I'm cutting out carbs."
- "I exercised today, so I deserve a reward."

Make a list of three messages *you tell yourself* that come from the diet mindset.

1. _____
2. _____
3. _____

While you may believe these phrases are helpful, take a moment to think about how you feel when you say them out loud or to yourself.

_____

_____

_____

Make a list of three messages *you've been given* by family, friends, health professionals, the media, and others who promote the diet mindset.

1. _____

2. _____

3. _____

How do you feel when these messages are directed at you?

_____

_____

_____

_____

Make a list of three messages *you give to others* that promote the diet mindset.

1. _____

2. _____

3. _____

Rejecting diet culture requires changing the messages you give (both to yourself and to others) and letting go of the messages you receive that come from a diet mindset. Use this awareness to notice when, where, and from whom you get these messages.

Rebound Eating

Rebound eating refers to eating that occurs in response to the deprivation caused by dieting, often resulting in physical and emotional discomfort. You may believe that when you're able to restrict certain foods for a time, that's how you're supposed to eat forever—and that when you override your restrictions it means you're lacking in willpower or doing something wrong. But what you're experiencing is actually a *natural* reaction to restriction.

When you tell yourself that certain foods are forbidden or off-limits, they increase in value, or "glitter," which can trigger rebound eating of those foods. Not giving your body enough nourishment during the day can also lead to rebound eating, especially at night.

In chapter 3, we'll look at the antidote to rebound eating, but for now, identify at least two foods (or food groups) that you currently try to limit for diet culture reasons—for example, to lose weight or because you think they're "bad" foods. (If you don't intentionally limit any specific foods for diet culture reasons, you'll soon learn why that's helpful!)

1. _____

2. _____

Chronic Dieting

The diet industry is a more than 70-billion-dollar business in the US alone that relies on the pressure people feel to have a thinner body. As a result, people try all kinds of methods to pursue weight loss. Unfortunately, the overwhelming majority of diets fail within five years, and people often end up at a higher weight than they began with. In fact, dieting is one of the biggest predictors of weight gain. While we want to be clear that there's absolutely nothing wrong with gaining weight or having a larger body, it's important to know that dieting often has the opposite effect of what it promises.

If you've tried to diet on multiple occasions, you are a chronic dieter. Ending this cycle is key to making peace with food and your body.

To begin, make a timeline of your experiences with dieting and note any instances of rebound eating:

FIRST DIET   *LAST OR CURRENT DIET*

⟵————————————————————————————————⟶

Now take some take to think about your experiences with the diet cycle by reflecting on or journaling about the following.

The reason I start a diet is:

_____

_____

_____

_____

The types of diets I've tried include:

_____

_____

_____

_____

When I break through my food restrictions (eat foods I'm not "supposed to" according to my diet), I feel:

_____

_____

_____

_____

Because of dieting, I've missed out on:

_____

_____

_____

_____

A Quick Look at the Research

Decades of studies have consistently shown that the vast majority of people who pursue weight loss will regain their lost weight.

- 1959: Albert Stunkard and Mavis McLaren-Hume review 30 years of data and conclude that diets are ineffective and that there is a 95 percent failure rate.

- 1992: The National Institutes of Health review weight loss programs and conclude that 90 to 95 percent of dieters regain weight, with one-third to two-thirds regaining weight within the first year and almost all regaining weight within five years.

- 2007: Traci Mann and colleagues review weight loss studies finding that weight reaches its lowest point around six months in, then starts increasing at about one year, after which weight regain speeds up over time. One-third to two-thirds of dieters end up higher than their pre-diet weight.

- 2015: Alison Fildes and colleagues conduct a study of over 278,000 people and find that the probability of dieters regaining all of their lost weight is between 95 and 98 percent.

Not much has changed over the decades, other than that the weight loss programs and plans are often using different language to sound more scientific or psychological. But still no proof exists that they can be sustained for more than a five-year period. While just about any diet works in the short run, by the one-year mark most people (who haven't already dropped out of a study) are regaining lost weight, and the rate of weight regain tends to increase over time. By five years, the vast majority of people have regained the weight they lost, if not more.

Imagine your doctor offered a medication that had a 5 percent chance of working. If you took it but didn't get better, would you blame yourself? And if you were then offered another medication with the same 5 percent chance of working, would you take it? If that also failed, would you continue to blame yourself? Understanding the rates of diet failure can help you let go of shame and guilt. You haven't failed your diet; your diet failed you!

Emotional Eating

If you describe yourself as an emotional eater, you may believe that's a problem. Let's start by acknowledging that eating is an emotional experience! Food can offer pleasure as you experience its taste and texture. Food can offer a sense of connection as you eat with your friends and family. Food can create feelings of gratitude as you feel nourished by the nutrients in the foods you consume.

Describe an eating experience that left you feeling pleasure, connection, or gratitude.

_____

_____

_____

_____

Nonetheless, if you believe that you're an emotional eater, you probably feel like you eat in response to all kinds of feelings: sadness, anger, loneliness, boredom—the list goes on and on. We'll explore ways to respond to the emotional aspects of eating in chapter 4. For now, we want to suggest that most people who consider themselves to be emotional eaters also experience deprivation due to dieting, which *increases* the chances that they will turn to food in times of distress. If you're caught in the diet cycle, it's hard to know for sure whether emotions are the driving force when you eat to the point of discomfort, or whether deprivation is actually the root cause.

Binge Eating Disorder

Binge eating disorder (BED) is characterized by frequent binge episodes, in which someone consumes large quantities of food in a short period of time and feels an accompanying lack of control during these episodes—this lack of control is a key feature of the disorder. People with BED come in all shapes and sizes, and people at the higher end of the weight spectrum do not necessarily have BED (you cannot tell anything about a person's relationship with food based on body size). Successful treatment of BED is not dependent on weight loss, a topic we'll address in chapter 5.

Although BED is relatively prevalent, it wasn't recognized as an eating disorder until 2013, when it was included in the fifth edition of the *Diagnostic and Statistical Manual of Mental Disorders* (DSM), which is used to diagnose mental health issues. The addition of BED to the DSM was an important step because it gave validity to this condition. Have you ever been told to just stop eating? To just put down your spoon or fork? These types of comments deny the reality of what people with BED experience.

If you binge, what have you been told—or what do you tell yourself—about how to end the binge?

_____

_____

_____

_____

If you have BED, your need to binge has become a way to survive in the world. You are not weak in character, lacking in willpower, or self-destructive. Instead, it's important to have compassion for the way in which eating became an adaptive strategy to make it through troubled times. After all, food is that earliest way we're soothed when we're born into this world. As Amy and her co-author Chevese Turner (Pershing & Turner, 2019) write in their book, *Binge Eating Disorder: The Journey to Recovery and Beyond*, "Problems with family or other significant relationships, significant losses, histories of emotional abuse, physical neglect, and sexual abuse are more correlated with BED than other eating disorders, and considerably higher than in the general population" (p. 14).

In chapter 5, we'll offer information to help you better understand BED and learn strategies to heal. Because the deprivation of dieting fuels binge eating, it is useful to look at the role of the diet cycle and rebound eating in your life. At the same time, turning to food in times of distress will likely still be an important coping mechanism that you use to help you survive, so be sure to go at your own pace and stay gentle with yourself.

Disordered Eating

Even if your eating behaviors don't constitute BED, you may still have what's known as *disordered eating*— problematic behaviors surrounding food that don't meet formal criteria for an eating disorder but that nevertheless cause significant distress. If you picked up this workbook, it's likely that you're hoping to have a more peaceful relationship with food. Here are some examples of behaviors that are typical of disordered eating. Which ones describe you?

- Skipping meals

- Overexercising (e.g., using exercise to punish yourself for eating "too much," getting upset if you have to miss a workout, continuing to exercise despite injury or illness)

- Fasting (intentionally going for long periods of time without eating, other than for a religious holiday, though it's also possible to approach religious fasts from a disordered mindset)

- Eliminating food groups without a legitimate medical reason (e.g., cutting out gluten if you don't have celiac disease)

- Feeling disconnected from your body's hunger and fullness cues

- Eating to the point of discomfort on a regular basis

- Dieting

- Feeling a sense of guilt or shame about your eating

Orthorexia

Orthorexia is a form of disordered eating that involves an obsession with "healthy" or "clean" eating. You may eliminate whole categories of foods or foods with specific ingredients, such as sugar or preservatives. While the focus isn't necessarily on weight loss, you become overly concerned about eating foods that you deem healthy, which gives you a virtuous feeling. As your preoccupation with eating in this way increases, you feel guilty if you stray away from this protocol, and your life may become more constricted. Orthorexia also negatively impacts mood and can make relationships difficult as you become increasingly isolated to maintain food rules.

The Cultural Backdrop

As you get ready to start healing your relationship with food and your body, let's take a moment to look more closely at the cultural backdrop in which the diet mindset is grounded. It's time to become more aware of what you've been taking in, and what you continue to take in, when it comes to messages about how to eat and how you should look—messages that come from all different forms of media. (We'll talk about how to deal with the people in your life promoting diet culture in chapter 9.) We wish there were a way to prevent diet culture messages from seeping in, or even bombarding you, but unfortunately that's not possible.

When you check out at the grocery store, chances are the magazines in the rack have the same themes: "Drop X pounds in four weeks! Lose weight and eat what you want! If I can do it, you can too!"

When January 1 rolls around, a slew of new books, written in scientific-sounding language, promise that you'll lose weight—and this time really keep it off for good!

On social media, influencers tout their latest "wellness" product or plan, making it seem that you can look like them if you buy what they're selling.

These messages play on both your fears and your hopes. If any of these so-called solutions actually worked—and by "worked," we mean that the plan or product would lead to sustainable weight loss not based on disordered eating behaviors—we wouldn't see them recycled over and over.

Although it's not possible to completely insulate yourself from diet culture, what *is* possible is for you to start to notice and reject the cultural messages that abound. Consider minimizing the number of messages you receive every day that are rooted in diet culture. For example, you might clear out any dieting books you have on your shelf, turn off TV commercials that promote weight loss, and delete social media accounts glorifying thinness.

Make a list of at least five sources of diet culture messages that currently exist in your life. For each one, note an action you can take and whether you feel ready at this time to take it:

Source of Message	Action I Can Take	Ready to Take Action?
1.		Yes or No
2.		Yes or No
3.		Yes or No
4.		Yes or No
5.		Yes or No

Cultural Subjectivity

Most of us have been taught to see the thinner body as the more attractive and healthier body, but cultural images of the ideal body change over time. Consider the following:

- When the United States was an agricultural economy, a heavier body was idealized because it meant that a family was successful in having enough resources to be well fed. With the advent of the Industrial Revolution and refrigeration, food was more plentiful, and at the same time, immigrants were coming to the US who were shorter and rounder. The cultural ideal changed to the taller, thinner body that is still revered today.

- During the Renaissance, fat bodies were praised and reflected in the paintings of the time. However, aesthetic ideals began to change with the rise of slavery and colonization in Europe, in which fatness became equated with "savagery." Sociologist Sabrina Strings explores these racial origins of fat phobia in her book *Fearing the Black Body*, where she describes how fatness was used as evidence of supposed out-of-control behaviors and racial inferiority in order to justify enslavement. She explains how fat phobia isn't about health, but rather a means of using the body to validate race, class, and gender prejudice.

To look at how body size standards have changed over the years, visit an art museum, look at an art book, or find famous artwork online. Notice the variety of shapes and sizes in the paintings and sculptures. How do you feel when you view these bodies?

_____

_____

_____

Diet Culture Is Sneaky

Because of the high failure rates of diets, many people, as well as commercial programs, agree that diets don't work. They have moved away from the language of "dieting," and have instead started to promote diets in disguise. These diets often take the form of wellness or health plans where food choices are manipulated for the purpose of weight loss.

Here are some examples of what you might hear other people say (or even say yourself):

- "It's a lifestyle program."

- "It's for my health."

- "It's part of my wellness plan."

Here are some examples of what you might hear companies advertise:

- "It's a change in mindset."

- "We offer a flexible eating plan."

- "It's not about weight loss."

While these programs masquerade as healthier alternatives to dieting, there are several pitfalls to these approaches. First, when you focus on metrics, such as calories, points, or the traffic light system of rating food (in which foods are ranked as green, yellow, or red based on their supposed healthfulness), it promotes food restrictions that can lead to disordered eating or eating disorders. Second, tracking food takes the pleasure out of eating and increases preoccupation with food and weight. Third, the continued focus on weight leads to shame if weight loss doesn't occur or if weight is regained. The blame is typically placed on the dieter, not the program.

These programs do not have any research to show that weight loss resulting from the plan is sustainable for the majority of participants. Remember, just about all diets work in the short run. But weight regain typically happens within a year and accelerates over time.

> " The diet industry is a virus, and viruses are smart. It has survived all these decades by adapting, but it's as dangerous as ever. . . . Dieting presents itself as wellness and clean eating, duping modern feminists to participate under the guise of health. Wellness influencers attract sponsorships and hundreds of thousands of followers on Instagram by tying before and after selfies to inspiring narratives. Go from sluggish to vibrant, insecure to confident, foggy-brained to cleareyed. But when you have to deprive, punish and isolate yourself to look 'good,' it is impossible to feel good. I was my sickest and loneliest when I appeared my healthiest. "
>
> —Jessica Knoll, *The New York Times*, June 8, 2019

There is nothing wrong with making choices about how to feed yourself in ways that support you physically and emotionally. But when the true purpose of those choices is to change your body size, you'll be subject to the same pitfalls as traditional diets. By taking weight out of the equation and focusing instead on foods that feel satisfying to your body and that offer the nourishment you need, you can cultivate a peaceful and satisfying relationship with food. No dieting required.

Imagine you felt at peace with food and your body. What would you do with that extra energy? Make a list.

_____

_____

_____

Clinician's Corner

This chapter focused on diet culture, diet failure, and the consequences that come from a diet mindset. If you are already familiar with an anti-diet approach and use this framework with your clients, we hope you'll find that the information offered in this chapter (as well as in the chapters to come) will validate and support your work with clients.

However, given that dieting is normative in our culture, the idea of rejecting diets may be new to you. The anti-diet philosophy is a paradigm shift, and you may find it challenging at times, especially if *you* are actively pursuing weight loss. We invite you to approach the remaining chapters with openness and curiosity as we explore the compelling reasons to let go of the diet mindset.

While you may not have received professional training around these issues, you've probably worked with clients who share concerns about their eating behaviors and body size. You may also have clients who come to you wanting to use an anti-diet approach to heal their relationship with food, even though this framework isn't familiar to you. We hope this workbook offers an opportunity to learn why more and more people are rejecting the diet mindset, and what to do instead.

Take a moment to reflect on the comments or responses you make in your work with clients that are reflective of the diet mindset.

_____

_____

_____

For now, increasing your awareness of how you bring diet culture to the clinical setting is a great place to start. In future chapters, we'll look at how to think about making a paradigm shift in your work with clients and discuss what to do when your clients are not ready or do not want to let go of the diet mindset.

CHAPTER 2

The Diet Cycle

We understand how hard you've tried to control your eating or lose weight by restricting your food intake in some way. While you may blame yourself for your "diet failure," there are strong psychological and physiological forces associated with deprivation that compel you to override these restraints. Understanding these forces is an important step in making peace with food.

The Psychological Effects of Deprivation

Imagine you're told that starting tomorrow, you can never have ice cream (or another pleasurable food that you believe is "bad") again. What would you do tonight?

If you responded that you would eat that food tonight, whether you're hungry for it or not—and eat more than you're hungry for—you're not alone.

A classic study by researchers at the University of Toronto looked at the impact of food restriction on cues for hunger and fullness (McFarlane et al., 1999). The researchers told the participants—some dieters and some non-dieters—that they'd be testing ice cream flavors. They were divided into three groups: The first group was given two milkshakes to drink before eating the ice cream, the second group was asked to drink one milkshake, and the third group was not given any milkshakes prior to the ice cream tasting. Here's what happened:

The non-dieters ate the most ice cream when they had not had any milkshakes, less ice cream when they had one milkshake, and the least amount of ice cream when they had two milkshakes.

In contrast, the dieters ate the least amount of ice cream when they had no milkshakes, more ice cream when they had one milkshake, and the most ice cream when they had two milkshakes.

What's happening here? With the diet mindset, you pass a point where you lose your restraint. In other words, you think, *What the heck! I've blown it anyway, so I might as well keep eating before I go back to my restrictions!*

We've known about this natural response for decades. In the mid-1940s, Ancel Keys was studying the effects of semi-starvation (Berg, 2000). He placed 36 conscientious objectors on a six-month diet that was adequate in vitamins, minerals, and protein. The men were allowed a caloric intake similar to many diets marketed by commercial weight loss programs today. As the men lost about 25 percent of their body weight, they experienced profound personality changes, becoming lethargic, irritable, distracted, apathetic, and depressed. They also became preoccupied with food, talking about it morning, afternoon, and night.

The food restrictions were lifted once the men entered the refeeding portion of the experiment. Free to eat what they wanted, the men engaged in binge eating for weeks yet continued to feel ravenous. The men's energy and emotional stability returned only after their weight was restored.

To reflect on how deprivation has affected you, write down three times when you've experienced the "what the heck!" effect and lost restraint when it comes to food.

1. _____

2. _____

3. _____

You may believe that when you're restricting food and feel "in control," you have a positive relationship with food. While you may be following the rules of diet culture, you're actually setting yourself up for the next binge or rebound eating episode. This is a natural reaction to deprivation, and it's not your fault. After being on a diet, it can take your body some time to recover, so please stay patient and compassionate with yourself.

The Physiological Effects of Deprivation

In our society, there is a common belief that with enough willpower, anyone can achieve the body type valued by diet culture. But this belief defies the physiology of weight regulation. Understanding the role of genetics, evolution, and adaptation will give you a stronger sense of why the pursuit of weight loss is doomed to fail in the long term for most people.

Genetics

Is your size and shape more a matter of nature or nurture? Research shows that nature is the more significant factor in determining your weight. When comparing identical twins who were raised apart, studies have found that both twins' body shape and size remain similar, even though they grew up in different environments (Stunkard et al., 1990). Another study compared weight gain among 12 pairs of twins who were given a significant number of extra calories and had to remain relatively sedentary over a four-month period. Within each pair of twins, the number of pounds gained and the distribution of fat was very closely matched. Likewise, when the twins were put on exercise regimes, the amount of weight lost varied among the sets of twins but was similar for each member of the pair (Bouchard et al., 1990).

The researchers have suggested that there's a form of "biological determinism" that makes people susceptible to weight gain. Or, as Judith and her co-author Ellen Frankel (Matz & Frankel, 2006) write in *The Diet Survivor's Handbook*, "Even if everybody ate the exact same foods and engaged in the same amount of daily activity, there would still be a wide variation of body sizes" (pp. 30–31).

If possible, reflect on the body shapes and sizes in your extended family or take a look at photos. Then consider the following:

What similarities and differences do you notice with your own body?

_____

_____

_____

_____

How were weight and shape viewed in your family?

_____

_____

_____

_____

How do those views impact you and your feelings about your body?

_____

_____

_____

_____

Evolution

Diets are framed as ways to lose fat, but they don't advertise the fact that you'll also lose muscle. Not only is muscle tissue important for helping your body move around, but it's also essential for the functioning of your heart, digestive system, and other major organs.

Your body also cannot tell the difference between a diet and a famine, causing it to go on high alert as you restrict your energy intake. After all, it has no way of knowing that you're trying to lose weight because it's the fashion of our time. Instead, your body thinks you're in trouble, and it does its best to keep you alive by slowing down your metabolism.

Think about our ancestors who lived in times of feast or famine. During times of feast, it was safe for the body to rev up and use lots of energy. But during times of famine, the body needed to slow down and hold on to every calorie. It was doing its job to manage its energy levels and keep our ancestors alive. The body gets better at storing fat after each period of starvation (or diet) in preparation for the next famine, so those whose bodies could adapt in this way were the ones who survived long enough to pass on their genes to future generations.

Diet culture sends the message that it's worth trying to diet no matter what. But what it doesn't tell you is that weight cycling changes the physiology of your body in a way that promotes long-term weight gain. While we want to be clear that there's absolutely nothing wrong with having a higher-weight body, it is important to understand that the very behavior you've been told will decrease weight tends to have the opposite effect. For example, research on former contestants of *The Biggest Loser* found that their metabolic rates were *permanently* lowered, so they had to eat significantly less food in order to maintain their pre-show weights (Kolata, 2016).

Many of our clients tell us that when they look back at photos of themselves when they were younger, they wish they could have felt content with the way they looked. "There was nothing wrong with me," said one of our clients as she looked at a picture of her 10-year-old self. "I had the body of my grandmother, strong and sturdy."

Consider taking a look through photos from earlier periods in your life as you reflect on the following questions.

When did you first decide that your body wasn't okay?

_____

_____

_____

_____

_____

As you look at a picture of yourself at that age when you first began disliking your body, how do you feel toward your younger self?

_____

_____

_____

_____

_____

If you could offer your younger self some compassionate words now, what would you say?

_____

_____

_____

_____

_____

Adaptation

Each of us has what's often referred to as a *set point*, which is really more of a set range of weights where our bodies naturally fall when we're able to eat enough to stay well nourished. Your set range is like a thermostat that adjusts according to the temperature: When it's cold, the heat kicks on, and when it warms up enough, the heat shuts off until the temperature drops again. Likewise, when you're eating enough, your metabolic rate increases and you have more energy, and when you're undereating, your metabolism slows down in order to conserve energy. Your weight regulation system works to keep your weight in the range that it's meant to be for you.

We've been taught to believe that our weight is under conscious control and that with enough willpower, we can decide our body's size. But numerous studies have challenged the idea that it's simply a matter of calories in and calories out (Bacon, 2010). While you may be able to "control" your intake and eat less than your body needs in the short term, you will find yourself eventually making up for the lack of nourishment whenever food is available. Remember, your body is interested in your survival!

If you find yourself at a higher weight than when you first started to diet, that's a natural, physiological phenomenon. As Glenn Gaesser (2002), author of *Big Fat Lies*, writes, "A number of studies have shown that the inescapable consequences of repetitive cycles of weight loss and gain appears to be ever-greater accumulations of fat" (p. 33).

It's *Not* Mind Over Matter

Now that you've learned about the psychological and physiological forces that drive you to override the effects of diet deprivation, we invite you to try a small experiment. When you're ready, begin to hold your breath. You can do it, right? As you keep going, notice what's happening. It's getting more difficult—and more difficult still. Although you can keep going for now, eventually you'll find yourself gasping for breath. Your body is going to keep you alive because, like we keep saying, that's its job!

Diets are similar. You can do it in the beginning, but it gets harder over time until your body rebels by increasing your hunger hormones, decreasing fullness hormones, lowering your metabolic rate, and triggering episodes of bingeing or rebound eating. (We also want to acknowledge that a small percentage of people have bodies that don't rebel, and instead they tend to develop eating disorders characterized only by restriction, such as the restricting subtype of anorexia nervosa.)

When you find yourself "losing control" of your eating after a diet, remember that it's actually a natural reaction to food deprivation.

The Diet Cycle

Let's take a deeper look at how the diet cycle works. While your story is unique, it's likely that it also follows this general pattern.

The Diet-Rebound Cycle

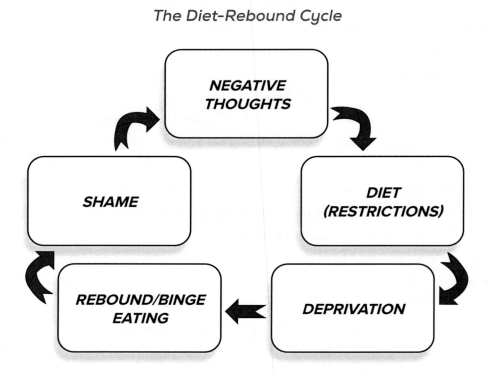

Negative Thoughts

Chances are that you don't begin your diet after having positive thoughts about yourself. Instead, you may bemoan the size of your belly or thighs, worry about your health, or have any number of negative thoughts about yourself and why you need to lose weight.

What are the negative thoughts that typically lead you to start your next diet? Make a list.

_____

_____

_____

_____

_____

_____

_____

_____

As you repeat these negative thoughts, it's natural that you want to take action to feel better about yourself. The solution typically offered by family, friends, health professionals, advertisements, and so forth is to pursue a program or plan that will change your body size and shape so that, in theory, you can feel more positively about yourself.

Diet (Restriction)

Once you decide to diet for weight loss, there are hundreds of plans and programs to choose from: low calorie, low carb, low fat. While the popularity of specific diet methods changes over time, at the time of this writing, intermittent fasting, keto diets, anti-inflammatory diets, and numerous commercial plans are in vogue. These diet plans are recycled and renamed over time, updated to sound more current and scientific even though they're built on the same old foundations.

Once you start your diet, there's a good chance you'll lose some weight because just about any program or plan works—in the short run. If you do lose weight, you may begin to get compliments from friends, family, coworkers, and health professionals like "I'm so proud of you," "You look fantastic," or "You're taking such good care of yourself."

Deprivation

If you did, in fact, receive compliments—and you liked the way they felt—then you might wonder why you, like most other dieters, didn't continue to stick to the plan or program. By now you likely also know the answer: The psychological and physiological deprivation that results from dieting sets you up to override whatever restraints you've put on yourself around food. This, in turn, leads to rebound or binge eating.

Rebound or Binge Eating

When you begin eating a lot after a diet to make up for the deprivation you've experienced, chances are that you're not turning to fruits and vegetables. Instead, you're likely eating the very foods that were forbidden as you pursued weight loss. These are the foods that now "glitter" for you, meaning that they increase in desirability. At the physiological level, your body also craves those energy-dense foods after a diet because it is trying to recover from the deficit and store as much energy as possible in preparation for the next "famine."

To consider how forbidden or restricted foods can trigger a rebound effect, complete the following prompts.

On my last diet, I restricted or didn't allow myself to eat:

_____

_____

_____

When I couldn't stick to my diet, I found myself eating:

_____

_____

_____

Reflect on the relationship between your responses.

If you notice any negative feelings arise, gently remind yourself that when you make certain foods "bad" or "forbidden," you increase the likelihood that these are the very foods you'll turn to when you feel compelled to override the restraints of your plan or program. This is a natural reaction to the food deprivation that comes from undernourishing your body—even if you refer to it as "healthy eating" or a "lifestyle change."

Up until now we've focused on the deprivation that comes from pursuing diets for weight loss. We also want to note that rebound eating can happen when you've experienced food insecurity, either in the past or in your current life. Any experience that forces your body to be deprived of the food it needs increases the likelihood of this response.

Shame

Once you engage in bingeing or rebound eating, you often feel shame for losing your "willpower" around food or for regaining any weight that you previously lost. Perhaps one of the most painful parts of the shame you might feel with weight regain is that the compliments stop. In the words of one former client, "When I regained the weight, everyone was silent. I felt heartbroken."

We believe that this feeling of shame is the most insidious part of the diet cycle. At its core, diet culture promotes body shame, as you're made to feel that there's something wrong with your body size, shape, or functioning. You try to follow the guidelines of diet culture by choosing a plan, whether it's an extreme diet or one considered to be moderate and "healthy," to lose the weight—and lose the shame. Yet as we've been pointing out, diets are doomed to fail for the vast majority. And who is blamed and shamed for the so-called failure? You! This leads the negative, body-shaming thoughts to return, and the diet cycle begins again—lasting years, or even decades. It's simply not fair.

As a chronic dieter, you've likely blamed yourself and experienced shame when you regained weight. If you could truly believe that the weight gain is not your fault—that you can't sustain weight loss from dieting—what would you say to yourself from a place of compassion?

_____

_____

_____

_____

Consider writing these words on a sticky note and placing it in a visible location. When you begin to have thoughts about starting a new diet, you might repeat these words to yourself to help break the cycle and remind yourself of your intentions to make peace with food and feel more at home in your body.

Understanding Shame and the Antidote to Shame

Let's take a deeper dive into the feelings of shame that typically accompany the diet cycle. Put a check mark by any of the following statements or feelings that resonate with you:*

Here are statements people make that are based in shame:

"I was bad today" (referring to what they ate).

"I'm embarrassed to go out at this size."

"I've let myself go."

"I'm ashamed to eat in public."

"I'm ashamed to be seen in public."

Here are feelings that people have that are based in shame:

"I feel that I am what I weigh and let the scale determine my worth."

"I envy thin people and equate their appearance with success, while my body implies failure."

"I feel 'less than' because of my body size."

"I feel that if only I could lose weight and get thin, all of these negative feelings would disappear."

Do you identify with any of these statements or feelings? If so, there's a very good reason. You live in a culture that promises that when you lose weight, you'll be happy, successful, attractive, and healthy. Given that higher-weight bodies are stigmatized in our culture, it makes sense that you might want to lose weight to be treated better—or, if you're already in a thinner body, that you would fear gaining weight. At the same time, you now know that diets ultimately don't work and, paradoxically, often lead to greater weight gain. We'll explore issues related to body image, health, and weight stigma in later chapters. For now, we want to give you some strategies to lessen your shame.

In her popular TEDx talk, *The Power of Vulnerability*, author Brené Brown explains how connection gives life meaning, and shame is a fear of disconnection. In other words, shame makes you wonder, *Is there something about me that makes me unworthy of connection?* While there are many reasons people can experience shame, two categories capture the underlying shame common to many of our clients: shame related to their appearance and body image, and shame related to being stereotyped or labeled. Sometimes we hear clients say, "I can feel fine in my body while I'm home, but as soon as I walk out the door I'm awash in shame." Their worry over how other people will judge their bodies interferes with any positive feelings they may experience in the safety of their own home.

---

* Reprinted from Matz & Frankel (2006) with permission of Sourcebooks.

Shame thrives on secrecy, silence, and judgment, meaning that the less you talk about it, the more control it has over your life. The antidote to shame is empathy. When you can share your story with someone who can listen to you with understanding and empathy, shame can't survive. The conundrum here is that there are generally few safe spaces to talk authentically about your struggles with food and weight without the backdrop of diet culture. Ironically, in diet culture, people constantly talk about dieting, weight, and out-of-control eating, but it's usually in the context of valuing the pursuit of weight loss.

As you consider being able to share your story, please complete the following:

The people I already talk to about the shame I feel around my eating or body image include:

_____

The people I can imagine feeling safe enough to talk about the shame I feel around my eating or body image include: _____

Right now, there is no one I can imagine feeling safe enough to talk about the shame I feel around my eating or body image.

Keep in mind that the more you can talk about your shame in the presence of supportive people, the more likely your shame will diminish. If you don't have an outlet to express your shame right now, consider some steps you can take to find or create a safe environment, which means that topics like calorie amounts, weights, and praise for weight loss are off-limits—there's plenty of that already in day-to-day diet culture conversations! We'll start you off with a few ideas, and you can add more as needed:

- Form a group of like-minded people who can go through this workbook with you.
- Start or join a monthly book club to read the multitude of resources related to intuitive eating, body acceptance, the experience of being higher weight, and so on.
- Join an online anti-diet or body positive community.
- Other ideas: _____

_____

_____

Shame resilience requires self-compassion. Stay compassionate with yourself as you gently move in the direction of letting go of the diet mindset and move toward healing.

Clinician's Corner

Increasingly, clients are seeking an anti-diet approach to heal their relationship with food and body shame. When a client comes to you who is already familiar with the pitfalls of the diet cycle, this chapter can validate their decision to let go of the diet mindset and help them process—and share with you—what they've experienced as the result of diet culture.

However, many clients will come to you saying, "I want to lose weight." When clients express this to you, how do you typically respond?

_____

_____

_____

Keep in mind that if you support your clients in dieting for weight loss or commend them for losing weight, if and when they regain the weight, their work with you may become another place where they feel like a failure. While your intentions to support them in their wish to be thinner likely come from a place of wanting to be helpful, unfortunately you will contribute to their shame.

No matter where you are in your own professional and personal journey, we encourage you to take a weight-inclusive stance that allows you to listen to your clients' experiences without judgment. This attitude helps build safety and trust as clients reflect on their own experiences with dieting and explore new strategies to make peace with food and their bodies.

Here are three scenarios to consider:

1. A new client comes to you stating they need to lose weight. You ask them to tell their story and, as they do, you respond to their situation with empathy. "I know how hard you've tried" or "I hear you're feeling scared right now" are responses that help build a connected relationship without you colluding in diet culture. Letting your client know that you hear their pain, that you understand how hard they've tried to lose weight, and that there are other strategies to support them when it comes to physical and emotional well-being offers them hope. As the client shares their story, you offer some of the information described in this chapter. Providing psychoeducation around diet failure, as well as new skills to heal their relationship with food, leaves most clients feeling hopeful.

2. You currently support clients in the pursuit of weight loss, but you want to make a shift away from promoting dieting behaviors. (It's okay to let clients know that while you've encouraged dieting in the past, as you've learned more about the research, you realize it's not the dieter's fault.) You explain that there are other solutions to help them make peace with food and their body and to support their physical and emotional health.

   Clinicians often find it helpful to be open and direct with their clients about this shift in mindset and to ask for permission to share what they're learning. For example, one therapist told his client, "I just attended a professional training on chronic dieting, and it's changing my way of thinking about food and weight. Would it be okay if I share some of the information I've learned?" If your client is open to hearing the information, together you can begin to explore the strategies offered in this workbook.

3. You've been working with a client to let go of the diet mindset, but at some point in your work together, they tell you they've decided to start another diet. Given the pressures to be thin in our culture, it's understandable that sometimes clients may feel the need to try to lose weight. You can remain supportive to your client as they explore whether their new plan is a viable option.

For example, after working together for over a year, one of Judith's clients announced she was starting a medically based weight loss program. Judith replied, "You know me well enough to know where I stand on the issue of dieting. At the same time, it's your body, and you get to decide what you believe is in your best interest. I'll be here to listen and, together, we can see how it goes." This nonjudgmental stance allowed her client to feel safe enough to describe the ups and downs of her latest weight loss plan. When it ultimately became unsustainable, they were able to process the diet failure and make sure the client didn't blame herself for the weight regain. Keep in mind that there's a difference between being supportive of clients who continue to pursue weight loss and supporting the actual behaviors (e.g., eliminating "forbidden" foods or overexercising).

Now that you've considered these three different scenarios, let's revisit the initial question we posed earlier, but with a slight change:

When clients come to you saying they want to lose weight, how would you like to respond?

_____

_____

_____

Given the pressures of diet culture, *you* may also struggle with chronic dieting, emotional or binge eating, or body shame. You may wonder if you can successfully help your clients with these issues if you haven't solved them for yourself. At this juncture, we'd like to emphasize that the essential factor is understanding that no matter how seductive diets may sound, the pursuit of weight loss almost always leads to weight regain, and often to physical and emotional harm. Unlearning diet culture takes time; you can still be an effective clinician as you work through your own relationship with food and with your body.

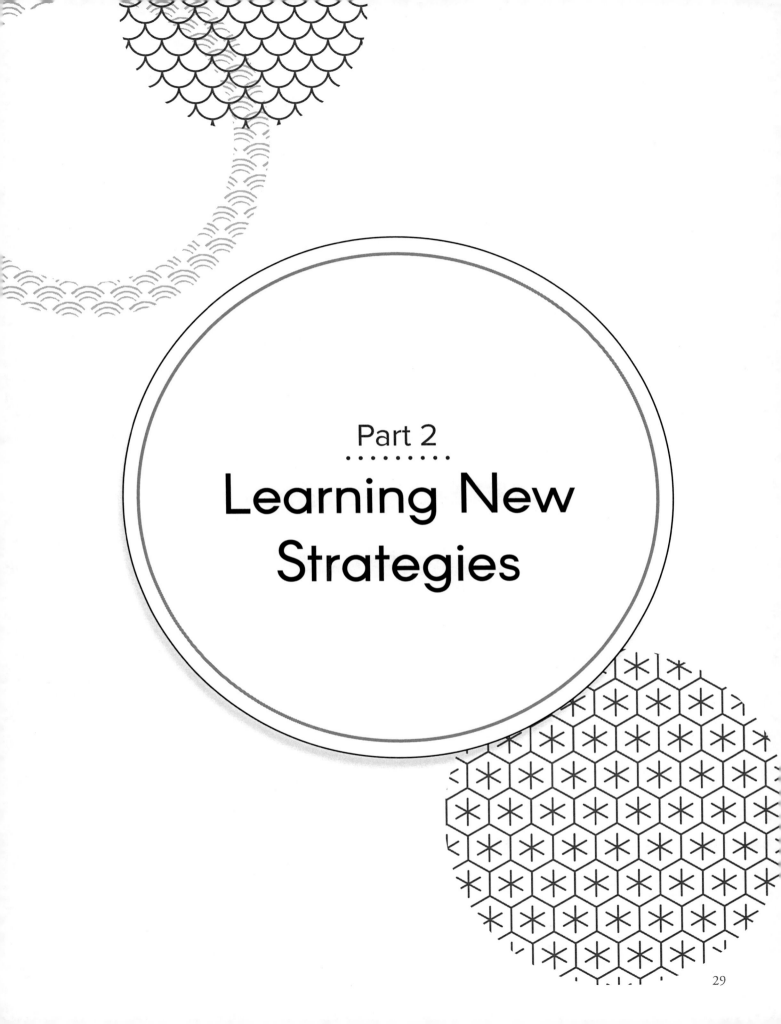

Part 2

Learning New
Strategies

CHAPTER 3

Attuned Eating—The Antidote to Dieting

Now that we've explored the problems with diet culture and the pitfalls of the diet cycle, it's time to take a look at how you can make peace with food. In this chapter, we introduce the guidelines of attuned eating, also known as intuitive eating. This approach offers a path to freedom from the diet mindset and supports you in eating for both nourishment and pleasure. Attuned eating guides you in feeding yourself based on your own needs and preferences when it comes to food. It is an antidote to the rebound eating that results from deprivation. (In the next chapter, we'll focus on how to address the emotional aspects of eating.)

To begin, take a moment to consider the different values underlying the diet mindset versus attuned eating. For each pair of words, circle the one that's most consistent with *your* set of values (the ones you truly believe in, not necessarily the ones you're practicing while on a diet).

Diet Mindset	Attuned Eating
Rigidity	Flexibility
Deprivation	Satisfaction
Guilt	Pleasure
Fear	Trust
External rules	Internal cues
Preoccupation	Empowerment
Weight loss goals	Nourishment
Shame	Compassion
Judgment	Acceptance
Constriction	Freedom
Feeling in control	Feeling in charge

Notice where most of your responses occurred. If they landed in the Attuned Eating column, you can be sure that the framework we're going to offer is full of behaviors and strategies to support your values!

Feeling in Control Versus Feeling in Charge

While many of the values underlying the diet mindset versus attuned eating are likely familiar to you, here's what we mean by the difference between *feeling in control* versus *feeling in charge.*

Imagine that you're at a party and are offered some birthday cake. You're in the midst of a restrictive plan of some sort, so even though the cake looks delicious, you decline. You feel deprived as you watch other people enjoy the cake, and it requires control to say no. But exerting that kind of control is like stretching a rubber band: Eventually, it snaps back. When you get home later that night—or sometime in the future—you make up for the deprivation you experienced by eating some of your "forbidden" foods, and as you do, you feel out of control.

Now imagine that you're at a party, and you're offered some birthday cake. You're hungry, you have some, and you enjoy it. Or you're not hungry and decline, with no sense of deprivation. Or you're not hungry, but you decide to have some anyway, with no guilt. These are all examples of being in charge.

Principles of Attuned Eating

Attuned eating guides you in deciding when, what, and how much to eat. Attuned eating helps you connect with and trust your body, rather than following someone else's rules. We understand how challenging that can feel at first. After all, diet and wellness culture constantly makes you feel that you can't be trusted to feed yourself. Based on our experience with thousands of people, as well as the research related to the harms of diets and the benefits of intuitive eating, we know that's not true. Sure, you'll run into plenty of challenges along the way; that's all part of the process. But we're here to help you figure out the mindset and strategies you need to create a more satisfying relationship with food. Let's begin!

When to Eat

Hunger is a bodily sensation that we're all born with. Babies cry when they're hungry, signaling that they need to be fed. A parent or caregiver offers a breast or bottle, and the baby eats, eventually turning away when satisfied. While there can be plenty of bumps in the road as everyone involved figures out the feeding relationship, the caregiver's response to the baby's physical hunger needs is at the core of this necessary task.

All kinds of things can interfere with innate hunger signals as this baby gets older. Schedules, lack of access to food, dieting, medical issues, and medications are some examples. For now, we're going to focus on how the pursuit of weight loss impacts hunger cues.

Think about your own hunger cues. How do you know when you're hungry? Make a list of any signals you experience. These can include physical sensations as well as thoughts and feelings. For each response, notice whether it's a comfortable or uncomfortable feeling.

1. _____ (comfortable or uncomfortable)

2. _____ (comfortable or uncomfortable)

3. _____ (comfortable or uncomfortable)

4. _____ (comfortable or uncomfortable)

5. _____ (comfortable or uncomfortable)

When we ask participants in our workshops to describe their hunger signals, common responses include a growling stomach, fatigue, headache, difficulty concentrating, irritability, a "hangry" feeling, weakness, dizziness, light-headedness, shakiness, nausea, an empty or gnawing feeling in the stomach, and persistent thoughts of food.

Many of these responses, such as headaches, weakness, and shakiness, indicate physical discomfort, meaning that you've likely waited too long to eat. Though your stomach may growl for reasons other than hunger (such as digestion), a growling stomach does tend to mean you're hungry—and for some people, it doesn't happen until they're at a relatively high level of hunger, if at all. Similarly, while thoughts of food can occur for many reasons (e.g., you're cooking or at the grocery store, or you see an ad on TV), they may be an indication that you need to eat.

However, diet culture encourages you to second-guess your hunger signals, to write them off as something else because you "shouldn't" be hungry. But attuned eating invites you to take these signals seriously and to nourish yourself when they arise.

Honoring Your Hunger

Using a rating scale for hunger can help you connect with your levels of hunger and fullness, though it may also be triggering for some people in recovery from disordered eating. If you're able to use the scale below to tune into your sensations of hunger without making rules about when you're "allowed" to eat, perhaps it can be a helpful tool. If not, feel free to skip the hunger scale. You might simply practice noticing and labeling your physical sensations of hunger instead.

1	2	3	4	5	6	7	8	9
Ravenous	Very hungry	Hungry	Somewhat hungry	Neutral	Somewhat full	Full	Very full	Extremely full

Keep in mind that when you're in a diet mindset, it's likely that at times you'll wait too long to eat, delaying until you're at a 1 or 2 on the hunger scale. When that happens, there's a good chance you'll make up for it by eating a lot later.

Think of a time when you were ravenous—it's happened to all of us!

How did it feel physically?

_____

_____

_____

_____

What kinds of foods did you crave?

_____

_____

_____

_____

After you finally did eat, what was your fullness level? _____

When you become too hungry, it's often a desperate feeling where you want to eat anything and everything. You're also likely to eat to a point of physical discomfort, which is common and completely understandable—your body is making up for lost time!

Instead, consider eating when you feel somewhat hungry or hungry—when your body is telling you it needs nourishment but before your hunger becomes overpowering. To get into this habit, practice checking in with your body every 15 to 30 minutes over the next few days, and notice whether you're experiencing any hunger signals. If it feels helpful, create a sticky note to remind you or set an alarm on your phone. If you're using the hunger scale, you might also note your level of hunger. When you notice any signs that you're hungry, move in the direction of eating soon after they arise, rather than pushing these signals aside.

Challenges to Honoring Your Hunger

Take a moment and practice checking in with your body right now. Are you hungry? Full? Neutral? Tuning in is an important step in reconnecting with your body. While it may sound simple, it may not be easy for all sorts of reasons. For example, you may have learned to suppress your hunger signals in order to avoid eating as you pursued weight loss. You may associate hunger with great discomfort because of your history of deprivation. You may have experienced trauma and disconnected from your body as a way to survive.

There are many reasons why you may have trouble connecting with your hunger. Put a check mark by any obstacles that apply to you. We've left additional room to add any other reasons that may affect your ability to experience hunger signals.

I'm not yet able to notice hunger until I'm ravenous.

Experiencing hunger of any kind makes me uncomfortable because of the distress I've experienced in the past from food insecurity or dieting.

I am neurodivergent and struggle to identify internal cues.

I have frequent binges or episodes of emotional eating, so I often don't get hungry.

My medication interferes with hunger cues.

I have a trauma history, and disconnecting from my body is still a way I survive.

Other: _____

_____

_____

Here are some possible ways to respond to each of these obstacles:

- *I'm not yet able to notice hunger until I'm ravenous.*
  - This is common for people with a history of chronic dieting. You've gotten used to suppressing your hunger signals, and it can take time to coax them back into awareness. You can help that process along by checking in with yourself frequently and with the intention of feeding yourself when hunger arises. As you consistently honor your hunger by eating, rather than pushing away the need for food as you did when restricting or dieting, you're likely to start noticing the cues before you become ravenous.

- *Experiencing hunger of any kind makes me uncomfortable because of the physical distress I've experienced in the past from food insecurity or dieting.*
  - It's understandable that if you've experienced the discomfort of hunger on a regular basis, you want to try to avoid that sensation. If you now have access to food—either because you're giving up restricting behaviors or because you currently have the resources to afford food—consider developing the following mantra: *I'll make sure I'm comfortably fed.* As you demonstrate to your body that you will feed it when it needs nourishment, it's likely that you'll feel safer in allowing the sensations of hunger to arise. Again, do your best to feed yourself before you feel very hungry or ravenous so that you can minimize discomfort.

    If you're currently experiencing food insecurity, it's completely understandable if noticing your hunger feels fraught. You might consider waiting to practice this principle of attuned eating and simply work on finding ways to get your food needs met as often as possible. Being able to eat when you're hungry is a foundational need and, we would argue, a fundamental human right. It's hard to focus on other things when that need isn't met.

- *I am neurodivergent and struggle to identify internal cues.*
  - If you're neurodivergent, you may not receive the bodily cues that reliably let you know you're hungry. Offering yourself food regularly throughout the day becomes essential in

making sure you get the nourishment you need. Attuned eating is flexible, and there's no rule that says you're *only* allowed to eat when you feel sensations of hunger. Eating according to a schedule rather than solely relying on internal cues may be an important tool to help you heal your relationship with food.

- *I have frequent binges or episodes of emotional eating, so I often don't get hungry.*

  ○ Food can be a source of comfort, which is a topic we'll address in chapters 4 and 5. Be patient with yourself as you work toward healing your relationship with food. If there is a moment that you can experience hunger, great! Try to notice how it feels to eat when you're hungry. At the same time, when you can't wait for physical cues, see if you can offer yourself some compassion: *I'm reaching for food, and I don't think I'm hungry. I look forward to the day when I'm able to experience more hunger signals.*

- *My medication interferes with hunger cues.*

  ○ Some medications can decrease appetite, while others increase it. If you are on any medications that suppress appetite, trying to eat solely in response to hunger cues will leave you undernourished; therefore, it's important to use other strategies, like offering yourself food regularly throughout the day. For medications that increase hunger, remind yourself that there is an important reason you're taking them, and let go of any shame that arises.

- *I have a trauma history, and disconnecting from my body is still a way I survive.*

  ○ If you've experienced trauma in the past or present, and especially if your body is the source of that trauma, you may tune out from bodily sensations to manage your distress. We'll take a deeper look at the effects of trauma in chapter 5. For now, do your best to let go of the diet mindset and to nourish your body throughout the day. As you find ways to heal your trauma, reconnecting with your body becomes more possible.

Challenges are to be expected, and each person's path toward peace with food will look different. Use this space to note any experiences with hunger cues that you want to explore further.

_____

_____

_____

_____

_____

_____

_____

_____

What to Eat

At the core of any diet or restrictive eating plan is a list of foods that you can and cannot eat, based on what's considered "good," "bad," "healthy," "unhealthy," "clean," or "dirty." As you follow these rules, you likely end up eating foods that don't actually satisfy you in the moment. You may also feel deprived because you can't eat foods that you desire.

When it comes to attuned eating, *you* get to decide which foods to eat based on your own individual desires and needs. If you're like most people, the idea of giving yourself permission to eat what you want feels both freeing and scary!

Think of a time you were hungry and ate exactly what you wanted. What adjectives would you use to describe how that felt?

_____

_____

_____

_____

Think of a time you were hungry but didn't eat what you wanted because you were dieting or restricting certain foods, you couldn't afford it, or it wasn't available. What adjectives would you use to describe how that felt?

_____

_____

_____

_____

When we ask this question to participants in our workshops, typical responses to the first question include: satisfied, content, happy, satiated, and joyful. Typical responses to the second question include: unsatisfied, deprived, frustrated, unfulfilled, disappointed, and still hungry.

When you allow yourself to make food choices that sound desirable to you, instead of following a rigid set of rules about "good" versus "bad" foods, you learn to trust your body and understand that satisfaction is key. This is the experience of an attuned eater. Day in and day out, they experience some physical hunger, choose foods that satisfy them, and then move on with their day until they're hungry again.

In contrast, people who are in the diet mindset usually find themselves preoccupied with thoughts of food throughout the day as they decide whether and what they should or shouldn't eat—and often don't end up physically or emotionally satisfied afterward. As one of our clients told us, "When I wake up in the morning, I decide if it's going to be a good day or a bad day when it comes to food. On a good day, I conform by eating what I'm supposed to on my food plan. On a bad day, I rebel and eat whatever I want. Either way, I'm miserable."

Imagine that instead of "following" or "breaking" a food plan, you were able to eat foods that satisfied you (to the extent they were available) most of the time. Use this space to write about how that would feel and what would be different in your life.

_____

_____

_____

_____

Making the Match

When it comes to eating, sometimes you'll hear people say about food, "That really hit the spot." We refer to this scenario as *making the match*, which is what happens when you eat what you're truly hungry for, instead of eating what you think you are "supposed" to eat. When you make the match, you feel both physically and psychologically satisfied.

The next time you're hungry, try tuning into your body and asking yourself what foods will satisfy you in this moment. See if you can determine what would both taste good *and* feel truly satiating, giving you a warm, relaxed feeling after eating—a pleasant sigh of having gotten what you wanted.

If you're not sure what will satisfy you, ask yourself: *Do I want something . . .*

- *Hot?*
- *Cold?*
- *Crunchy?*
- *Soft?*
- *Smooth?*
- *Salty?*
- *Spicy?*
- *Sweet?*
- *Bland?*
- *Substantial?*
- *Refreshing?*

Of course, it's impossible to get exactly what you want every time you're hungry. Given your circumstances, you can do your best to get what you desire or as close to it as you can. For example, let's say you get home from work and realize you'd like some lasagna. But you don't have the ingredients—or even if you do, by the time you could prepare it, you'd be ravenous. Maybe you decide to make some other kind of pasta instead, as you have some spaghetti and a jar of sauce in your pantry that would be quick to prepare. You also have some parmesan cheese in the refrigerator that you can sprinkle on top—a good enough match!

Or perhaps you realize that you want that melted cheese to feel satisfied. You prepare a grilled cheese and tomato sandwich instead—close enough!

Given this experience, maybe you plan to buy the ingredients for lasagna the next time you're at the grocery store so that in the future, you have what you need. You might cook it when you have the time and then freeze it so you can microwave it in the future when it will hit the spot. Or you might buy frozen lasagna to keep on hand. If you're in a position to do so, maybe you decide that you want it badly enough that night to order it from a local Italian restaurant. There's no right or wrong here—it's always up to you to decide how to best honor your needs and nourish your body.

We also want to acknowledge that the cost of food influences what you're able to provide yourself. Attuned eating is flexible, and you can adapt it to meet your circumstances. Most importantly, you can let go of the diet mindset and choose foods—without guilt—that help you feel as satisfied as possible.

Making the Match

Erica had a cup of coffee before joining a virtual webinar to learn more about attuned eating. She volunteered to work with Judith to figure out what she was truly hungry for.

Judith: If your fairy godmother were going to appear at your door to bring you exactly what you want to eat, do you know what she'd bring you?

Erica: I have a protein bar with me. I usually like that in the morning.

Judith: When you think about eating the protein bar, does that feel like it will satisfy you?

Erica: Not really.

Judith: Let's start with temperature. That's often the easiest to identify. Can you tell if you want something hot or cold?

Erica: Definitely hot.

Judith: Hot and soft, or hot and more solid?

Erica: I think soft would be good.

Judith: Soft like soup or soft like oatmeal?

Erica: I think I need some protein. Soft like eggs.

Judith: Eggs, that's great. How do you want your eggs prepared? Scrambled, sunny side up?

Erica: An omelet sounds really good.

Judith: What would you like in your omelet?

Erica: I want some cheese.

Judith: What kind of cheese? And any other fillings?

Erica: I'd like some cheddar cheese with mushrooms and spinach.

Judith: Is there anything else you'd like with your omelet? Some toast or fruit?

Erica: I'd like a piece of toast. I really like melon this time of year, and I think I have some cantaloupe.

Judith: Take a moment and think about what you've come up with as satisfying: a mushroom, spinach, and cheese omelet with toast and some cantaloupe. When you think about how that would taste and feel in your body, what do you think?

Erica: It would be awesome.

Judith: That's a lot different from a protein bar.

Erica: Yeah. That's what I usually allow myself. I don't even think about whether I want something else.

Fortunately, Erica had the ingredients she needed to make the meal she desired, and she reported later in the day that it felt great. But even if she didn't have the exact ingredients, by checking in with herself, she could have gotten much closer to what would satisfy her. If she didn't have the veggies she desired, she still could have used eggs and cheese to make an omelet. Even if she didn't have any of those ingredients, she would still know that she wanted something hot and savory—definitely not the protein bar. By tuning in, she'd be more likely to choose foods that would feel satisfying, which is key to helping her heal her relationship with food.

If making the match is a new skill for you, it can take time to figure it out. That's okay. It's not about getting it right or wrong. Instead, think about conducting mini experiments. After you eat, you can reflect on whether you truly made the match. If so, play it up for yourself by acknowledging how good it felt. If not, ask yourself what would have made it better. For example, perhaps you needed fries with your burger because something was missing, or you would have preferred a burrito bowl instead of a burrito because you didn't like the texture of the tortilla.

The next time you're hungry, slow down and tune into your body. Ask yourself what would satisfy your hunger, and do your best to come as close as you can, given what's available to you. When you're done eating, describe the experience here.

When I was hungry, I chose to eat: _____

_____

If it felt satisfying, take a moment to notice the way you feel. Play it up to yourself—*I made a match and it feels:*

_____

_____

_____

_____

_____

If it didn't feel satisfying, ask yourself what would have made it feel better. Use this space to write down the feedback your body gave you that will help you the next time you feel hungry.

_____

_____

_____

_____

_____

Novelty Versus Habituation

There's a high probability that when you think of eating what you're hungry for, you feel some fear. That's understandable, given that you've been told over and over that you can't be trusted with food. You likely find that when your "glitter" foods are around, it takes a lot of energy to keep yourself from eating them. Or you end up eating them in a way that feels out of control. The reality is that the foods you've put off-limits have *increased* in value because you've kept them scarce, and we know that scarcity makes us anxious.

Imagine that you receive a text from your utility company saying that your water is going to be shut off in 30 minutes. What would you think about? What actions would you take?

Chances are you weren't thinking about water a minute ago. If you typically have water available at all times, you probably don't think much about it unless you become thirsty or need it for another purpose. When you get so used to something being around that it no longer has much meaning or allure for you, this is called *habituation*. You habituate to what is consistently present in your environment. In contrast, when something is restricted, it becomes more *novel*. You start to be much more aware of its presence, and you attach greater meaning to it.

That means that when you realize your water will soon be taken away, your anxiety about having water likely increases. You might start to fill containers with water, take a shower, or run to the grocery store to buy bottled water. This change in anxiety and preoccupation with water is similar to the anxiety and preoccupation you experience, day in and day out, when you deprive yourself of particular foods.

Think about the foods in your kitchen to which you are habituated. You don't think much about them, and maybe you even forget that they're there. But when you're hungry for them, you're glad to have them available.

Now, think about the foods you like but don't usually have in your home. Perhaps one day you buy them at the grocery store on a whim or someone brings them to your home. It's hard to forget they're there. They "call" to you from the pantry or fridge. You spend time deliberating about whether to have some. You use control to avoid eating them, or you "give in" and eat them in a way that perhaps feels out of control. It creates anxiety to know that they're in your house.

In contrast, when you keep foods consistently available—with permission to eat them—they lose their novelty. The idea of bringing these foods into your home may feel scary, exciting, or both. Here are some strategies to help you get started:

Make a list of your feared or forbidden foods, and rate them from least to most challenging.

1. _____

2. _____

3. _____

4. _____

5. _____

Pick one of the least challenging foods that's available to you, and buy and eat as much of it as you want for the next week or two. Notice how your relationship with that food changes over time, and continue making it available to yourself as often as you want after the end of this experiment. Then repeat this process with other foods on your list as you feel ready.

We always want to encourage you to move at your own pace. If you don't feel ready to buy your feared foods, consider trying this visualization: Choose a food that you think would be hard to stop eating once you started. Now imagine that you're going to have it—and only it—for breakfast, lunch, and dinner for the next month.

Notice whether anything changes in the way you feel toward that food.

People often find that their desire for that food diminishes over time. They notice that there are other foods they want instead. Sometimes people will say, "Oh, I get it! I'll get so sick of it I'll never want it again!" But the goal isn't to make you "sick" of any food. Instead, you're learning to put the food in its proper place—it's there for you when you want it, when it's a good match for your needs. At the same time, it's not the *only* food you'll want.

The core message here is that all foods fit! We've never met anyone who, when all foods are available without stigma or shame, *only* wants cake, candy, ice cream, chips, or whatever else diet culture considers to be "bad" foods. We've also never met anyone who, when listening to their body, *only* wants salads, veggies, fruit, and protein. We need variety, and we can learn to trust our desires to lead us there.

To give you an example of how habituation can look in practice, let us introduce you to Evan, who felt ready to try making peace with one of his feared foods: potato chips. He usually avoided them, but they were always in the house for his children to have with their sandwiches. Sometimes at night, Evan would find himself taking out the bag and eating them in a way that felt out of control. He acknowledged that he would also enjoy chips with his sandwiches, although he preferred different kinds of chips than his kids did.

Evan wanted to allow himself to eat potato chips when they were a good match for his hunger—and to be able to do this for the rest of his life! The next time he went to the grocery store, he was pleased to find that his favorite brand was on sale, and he bought about five or six bags for himself.

Not surprisingly, when Evan first got the chips, it was exciting. He wanted to eat them often, and he did. Yet over a short period of time, they began to lose their glitter. He soon found that while he did enjoy having chips with his sandwich and was glad to have them available, he no longer felt compelled to binge on them at night.

Here are the actions that Evan took that helped him make peace with chips:

- He no longer let himself get too hungry.

- He gave himself permission to eat chips whenever he wanted them, without judgment.

- He never let them run out and, as a result, became habituated to them.

- He checked in with himself about making the match and discovered that he typically enjoyed them with a sandwich.

Now, Evan sometimes even forgets the chips are in the pantry—something he hadn't believed was possible. Of course, the goal of habituation isn't to forget about your previously feared foods and stop eating them; it's to help them take their rightful place as just one option among many foods that you eat and enjoy whenever you want.

Now it's your turn! Use this space to write about your experiences with habituation. Keep in mind that we are focusing on healing your rebound eating due to food restrictions or undernourishing your body. You may still need to turn to food for emotional reasons, which we will explore in the next chapter.

_____

_____

_____

_____

_____

_____

Undoing Diet Patterns

It takes time to let go of the messages you've internalized about when and what you're supposed to eat. Here are a few more strategies to support you in making peace with food.

Semantics Matter

It's common to hear people say, "I was good today" or "I've been bad this week," referring to what they ate. This language is part of diet culture and the moral judgment that it places on food.

Instead of using value judgments to describe your eating experiences, try simply tuning in and noticing whether your eating experiences feel satisfying or unsatisfying. Keep in mind that the same foods can feel satisfying or unsatisfying at different times. For example, pizza might feel just right when you need something warm and cheesy, but totally unfulfilling when you want something crunchy and refreshing. A salad with chopped veggies and chicken might be a good match in that case, but it can feel deeply unsatisfying when what you really want is something warm and hearty.

Take a moment to review your eating experiences for today, noticing when you felt satisfied and unsatisfied.

I felt satisfied when I ate:

_____

_____

_____

_____

I felt unsatisfied when I ate:

_____

_____

_____

_____

Practicing these sentences will help you shift away from diet culture as you change the way you talk to yourself about the types of foods you eat.

Choosing Former Diet Foods

Many people find that once they stop dieting, there are certain foods that make them feel like they're still on a diet. Let's say you ate apples because you were "supposed" to, but you don't really like them. You might decide that the fruits you really enjoy are bananas and berries, and that you no longer want to eat apples. That's fine!

Now let's say you really do like apples, but every time you think about eating them you associate it with being on a diet. As a result, you may avoid them. Think about how to let go of the diet mindset so you can truly decide for yourself if a particular food gives you pleasure.

Use this space to make a list of foods that make you feel like you're on a diet.

_____

_____

_____

_____

_____

Next, use your senses and imagination to consider the taste, texture, smell, and color of each food. Does anything about it appeal to you? If so, give yourself permission to eat it when it's the right match for you in a given moment. Notice whether it gives you satisfaction, and if so, you can reclaim that food as a source of nourishment and pleasure.

Keeping Food Available

Imagine a parent is out for the day with their toddler. The child is hungry and starts to cry. The parent responds, "It's okay, honey. We'll be home in four hours, and then I'll get you something to eat." The parent likely wouldn't do that because the toddler would be miserable—and so would the parent!

But we often hear from clients that they went out in the morning to do an errand, which turned into more errands. Hours later, they came home ravenous. Or they planned to go out for lunch at work but couldn't get away because of an unexpected meeting, leading them to get too hungry.

Just as parents or caregivers bring snacks with them when they're out with young children, think about keeping food with you. You can put snacks in a lunchbox, a bag, a backpack, or whatever container is convenient. The foods you put in your container can be anything you might desire during the day.

Imagine you're planning to bring food with you over the course of a day. What would you include?

_____

_____

_____

_____

Use these responses to support you in experimenting with keeping food available to the extent possible given your circumstances.

It's a Family Affair

As you focus on choosing foods that bring you satisfaction, you may wonder what that means for family meals, especially if you're the one who prepares food for others. Does everyone get to decide exactly what they want for dinner? We want to assure you that you're not expected to be a short-order cook!

Instead, meals with lots of variety generally ensure that everyone can find something they'll enjoy. Maybe someone at the table likes the salad, bread, and spaghetti, but not the meatballs or fruit, while someone else chooses to eat the spaghetti, meatballs, and fruit but doesn't want the salad or bread. Or let's say you're in the mood for tacos with beans and rice, while your partner decides they'd rather heat up last night's stir-fried chicken and veggies. Are you okay with the idea that you can each eat different foods and still feel connected?

Families have different ways of managing mealtimes, and there's no one right way. Sometimes people need to eat at different times due to work or school schedules. Food choices may be limited due to budget. Attuned eating is flexible, and feeding a family as well as yourself requires some time and energy.

If you live with other people, write down some strategies to support the differing food needs of each individual, without becoming burdensome to those preparing the food.

_____

_____

_____

_____

_____

_____

_____

Social Situations

If you're meeting friends for a meal at 6:30 p.m., and you're hungry at 5:00 p.m., what should you do? You know that when you get overly hungry, you feel deprived and anxious, and it also makes you more likely to eat to discomfort. At the same time, you don't want to eat a whole dinner now and have no appetite for the food at the restaurant.

In situations like this, it can be helpful to think about "arranging" your hunger. You know that you want to be hungry, but not ravenous, when you meet your friends, so you decide to have something to eat now that will help tide you over until 6:30 p.m. What will give you some satisfaction now but leave you ready for your dinner? As always, there's no universally right answer. Maybe in this moment it's some popcorn or nuts, some fruit, a cookie and milk, some chips and hummus, or a slice of leftover pizza. You get to decide!

Now when you get to the restaurant, you can have the satisfaction of eating a delicious meal with friends, without having deprived yourself in advance.

The next time you're in a situation where you plan to eat at a certain time but get hungry sooner, experiment with "arranging" your hunger so that it comes back at the designated time, while also satisfying it now. Write about your experience here.

_____

_____

_____

_____

_____

Eating Styles

Beyond nourishment and pleasure, food has all kinds of other meanings in our lives. Your values, religious practices, cultural traditions, and health concerns are examples of other aspects of your relationship with food.

Values

You may have philosophical reasons for eating or avoiding certain foods. For example, you may be vegetarian or vegan, choosing to eliminate meat and other animal products from the foods you consume. Attuned eating is flexible, and choosing what to eat based on your values is compatible with the concept of "making the match" as you match with your beliefs.

At the same time, it's important to make sure your choices aren't guided by the diet mindset. We know of people who realized they became vegetarian because they believed meat products were "too fattening" or not "clean," and with this awareness they decided to add them back in as food options.

If you adopt a vegan diet because of philosophical beliefs, pay attention to whether you're restricting food at some level. For example, items such as Oreo cookies and French fries—foods that are often off-limits on diet plans—are vegan. Do you give yourself permission to eat vegan foods that also contain sugar or fat?

We also want to note that within the vegan community, there's often an emphasis on having a thinner body. This body shaming can be stressful if you want to be vegan while working to let go of the diet mindset and feel more at home in your body. As always, finding people who are supportive of your efforts will be of great help to you.

Religious Practices

You may follow certain dietary guidelines, such as a Kosher or Halal diet, due to the practices of your religion. Again, eating in a way that reflects your religious beliefs is consistent with attuned eating. There are also times that you may fast or give up certain foods as part of your religion, such as Yom Kippur if you're Jewish, Lent if you're Christian, or Ramadan if you're Muslim. If these practices are part of the way you restrict food due to an eating disorder, or if they trigger eating struggles, find out whether your religion allows for flexibility in skipping these practices at this time.

Cultural Traditions

Food is an important part of your cultural heritage that can connect you to your family, community, and history. Have you avoided some of these foods because they didn't fit into the restrictions dictated by diet culture? If so, it's time to give yourself permission to eat them again in a manner that nourishes you. Conversely, you may have grown up in a family where food is a way of expressing love, and turning down offers of more food is experienced as a sign of rejection. As you reconnect with your own hunger signals, it's up to you to decide how to navigate these expectations.

Health Concerns

People often identify health concerns as one of the biggest reasons they restrict certain foods. This may be a more general health-related belief, such as the belief that eating sugar is "bad," or it may be in response to a specific health condition. In chapters 7 and 8, we'll look at myths around food and health as well as how to make decisions about food choices to support your body when you have a specific concern. For now, we want to reassure you that attuned eating supports people with all types of health issues. In fact, we've found that when people end the deprivation that comes from dieting, they're actually in a stronger position to make use of nutrition recommendations if they do develop a health condition where food choices may have an effect.

For example, someone with constipation may decide to add fiber to help their system. While they may have cut out carbs as part of a diet plan, they're now in a position to add back grains, including whole grains, to their intake, if those are foods they enjoy. Clients with diabetes can learn to test their blood sugar after eating to learn how different foods affect them, allowing them to find ways to eat what they enjoy while supporting their bodies without following a rigid food plan.

Use this space to reflect on how these aspects of eating, as well as any other aspects that we haven't already mentioned, impact your relationship with food.

_____

_____

_____

_____

_____

_____

Is Food Addiction a Real Thing?

When Christy was struggling with disordered eating, she was convinced she was "addicted" to food—specifically high-carbohydrate, sugary, and often high-fat foods. She couldn't bring them into the house without eating them in a way that felt totally out of control, polishing off entire boxes of cereal and bags of cookies and chips far faster than she cared to admit to anyone. She wanted to stop eating these foods but was utterly incapable of doing so, leading her to believe that she had an addiction.

The concept of food addiction is problematic. As we've discussed, restriction and deprivation cause certain foods to "glitter"—to have an almost irresistible appeal that drives us to consume them in a way that might feel compulsive and out of control. While those foods can certainly seem addictive, in reality the term *food addiction* is a misnomer. In fact, the culprit is the *restriction*—not the foods themselves.

Numerous research studies on so-called food addiction have found that "addictive" behaviors only occur in the context of deprivation—specifically intermittent, restricted access to high-sugar or high-fat foods (sometimes along with restricted access to food overall), as opposed to consistent access to all kinds of foods (Muñoz-Escobar et al., 2019; Westwater et al., 2016). One study found that teens who were restricting foods and then exposed to pictures of highly palatable foods had greater brain activity compared to teens who were not restricting, concluding that calorie restriction increases the brain's attention to and the reward value of the very foods that have been restricted (Stice et al., 2013).

The research has not found any convincing evidence that food contains substances that are truly addictive in the way that drugs and alcohol are. Granted, it might feel like if you let certain foods pass your lips you can't stop eating them, or that if you have them in your cupboard you will keep going back for more. It might feel like these foods are completely irresistible, even when you're already full. Those feelings are very real, but they're not caused by true addiction. Even though the way you're eating them might *feel* addictive, it's actually restriction and deprivation driving that feeling.

How Much to Eat

If you've followed diets in the past, you've probably been told the amount you should eat. Whether it was based on measuring out food, counting calories, or calculating points, the decision about how much to eat came from an external source.

With attuned eating, internal cues become your main source of information in deciding how much to eat, along with your circumstances, such as how much food is available. *You* get to decide how you want to feel when you're finished.

Earlier in this chapter, we focused on the "hunger" side of the hunger scale. Now it's time to look at signs of fullness. As mentioned earlier, if you find it distressing to think about rating your fullness on a scale, feel free to skip this activity. You might try simply noticing the physical sensations of fullness instead, though that can still be upsetting for some people in recovery from various forms of disordered eating. If focusing on fullness doesn't work for you at this point, you can continue to practice noticing and honoring your hunger signals, with the awareness that feelings of fullness may become easier to tolerate when you're no longer suppressing hunger.

1	2	3	4	5	6	7	8	9
Ravenous	Very hungry	Hungry	Somewhat hungry	Neutral	Somewhat full	Full	Very full	Extremely full

If you are using the fullness scale, take a moment to reflect on how you like to feel after you've eaten. Now, think about how you tend to actually feel after you've eaten.

Many people who engage in rebound or binge eating often find themselves in the "very full" or "extremely full" region of the hunger scale, and they usually report physical discomfort. This is a common and perfectly understandable response to deprivation: If you often eat less than you want and need, your body tends to drive you to eat to the point of discomfort to make up for the deprivation. Over time, as you start honoring your hunger more consistently—and trust that you won't deprive yourself of the foods you enjoy—you'll likely find that your fullness doesn't reach those extreme levels as often.

Remember to AIM

When deciding how much to eat, a helpful tool to honor your fullness is to remember to AIM. This acronym stands for attunement, intention, and mindfulness.

- **Attunement:** The strategies you've learned so far in this chapter are about attunement. When you ask yourself, *Am I hungry?* and *What would be the best match for my hunger?* you've attuned to your hunger needs. This process helps you reconnect to your body and increase satisfaction when you eat.

- **Intention:** Before you eat, consider how you want to feel on the fullness scale when you're done eating—and the amount of food you think you'll need to get there. At the end of the meal, check in with your body without judgment, and notice whether you're at the level of fullness you wanted to be. If you need more food, have it! If you're at a higher level of fullness than you'd intended, consider whether you were actually hungrier than you'd thought, if you'd been deprived of food (either intentionally or unintentionally), or if there were any other subtle forms of restriction that may have driven you to eat more. Practicing this strategy can help strengthen your mind-body connection.

- **Mindfulness:** In general, mindfulness is a practice of being aware of what's happening in the present moment, without judgment. Applying this concept to eating means letting go of thoughts that interfere with your ability to be present with food, such as calculating calories or points, or thinking about whether you're "allowed" to eat a particular food. Instead, you can notice the way food tastes and feels in your body, without judgment.

  Mindfulness is a practice that can help support attuned eating, but in diet culture, it unfortunately tends to get twisted into a diet rule. You may have engaged in a mindful eating experiment where you ate a raisin or an orange slice very slowly, noticing all that you could about its flavor and texture as you kept it in your mouth over a period of time. This experience can potentially be useful in reminding you to savor your food and enjoy the pleasure it brings, but it certainly isn't a practical way to feed yourself! You don't need to eat like that on a regular basis (or at all) in order to practice mindfulness with food. People also eat at different paces—some of us eat more slowly and some faster—and that's okay. You might simply aim to use mindfulness to help you notice and enjoy the pleasure that comes from eating, without being rigid about it.

To understand how using AIM can affect your eating experience, think of a time when you told yourself you shouldn't eat something but then decided to have some anyway. Perhaps you initially wanted just to have a bite or two but then had some more. You might have been eating directly out of the bag or carton, and before you knew it, you had eaten to the point of extreme fullness. Use this space to describe how that experience felt physically and emotionally.

_____

_____

_____

_____

_____

Now, imagine that you had given yourself permission to eat whatever it was you were wanting (*attunement*) and that you checked in with your body to decide how much you needed to feel satisfied (*intention*). You took that amount and put it on a plate or in a bowl, sat down with full permission to eat it, savored the taste, and noticed how it felt in your body, returning for more if desired—again with full permission and without judgment (*mindfulness*). Use this space to describe how that experience would have felt physically and emotionally.

_____

_____

_____

_____

_____

Distractions

To help you stay connected to your body and truly feel your fullness cues, it can be helpful to practice eating without the distraction of the TV, computer, or smartphone—this is part of eating mindfully. Yet there are all kinds of reasons why you may not be able to turn your full focus on the eating experience. You may live with family or have roommates and when you eat together, you're engaged in conversation. That's a good thing! You can still take a moment here and there to check in with your body and notice how it's feeling.

Or you may live alone, and it may feel too quiet to eat without distraction. Perhaps you turn on some music or a podcast or find another way to create the environment that feels right for you. Mindful eating doesn't mean that every meal and snack has to be eaten in silence with full attention on the food; expecting that of yourself would be rigid and impractical. The key is simply to pay some attention to your internal cues for hunger, fullness, and satiation, in the context of whatever else is going on while you eat.

If you've experienced trauma, the process of slowing down and tuning into your body may not be accessible at this time. You may need distractions while you eat, and that's okay. This is a process that looks different for everyone. Over time, attuned eating can help you reconnect in a safer way with your body. Expect it to take time. We'll take a deeper look at eating and trauma in chapter 5.

Mindful Eating and Flexibility

Cassandra recently set some boundaries in her workplace so that she would have enough time to eat without being on the computer at the same time. It felt so much more satisfying to eat with awareness and to appreciate the way her meal tasted and felt in her body, while also having a chance to chat with her coworkers in the break room or text with her friends. On Friday, she had a doctor's appointment during her lunchtime. She knew that if she ate her meal mindfully, she would be late for her appointment. But if she didn't eat before she left, she would end up ravenous. Cassandra took her lunch with her and ate it in the car. While it wasn't her preferred way to feed herself, this flexibility meant she could take care of the multiple needs she had that day.

Helpful Phrases to Honor Fullness

One way to learn how to trust your fullness cues is to repeat certain phrases to yourself before, during, or after an eating experience. As you read through these phrases, remember that they're strategies to support you in moving toward healing your relationship with food. They are dependent on your own individual circumstances regarding access to food, and they are not meant to be used as new rules or sources of judgment that lead to self-criticism. Instead, keep them in mind and notice if they help you change your relationship with food over time. After each phrase, use the space provided to reflect on how it feels to you.

If I stop now, I can have it again when I'm hungry.

When you eat your restricted foods, there's a good chance that you tell yourself, *Now that I've eaten the cookies* (or whatever is forbidden for you), *I might as well keep eating because starting tomorrow* (or Monday, or January 1) *I can't have it anymore.* The belief that these foods are going away typically compels you to keep eating them.

Once you embrace the idea that all foods fit and that you're not going to take anything away, it becomes safe to stop. If you're eating some pizza and notice you're satiated, you can remind yourself that you'll be able to have pizza again whenever you want, including later that same day if you feel like it. When you truly believe that the food isn't going away, you're likely to find that the incentive to eat to the point of discomfort diminishes.

How does this feel to you?

_____

_____

_____

_____

_____

I'm full but not satisfied. What would have felt better in my body?

You may find that, at times, you feel full, but there's something missing. This might happen when you eat something that doesn't truly "hit the spot," such as a salad when you really desire a sandwich, because you want to follow your food rules. As a result, you may find yourself still searching for something to satisfy you. As you try to fill that hunger need, you may end up at an uncomfortable level of fullness.

Instead of criticizing yourself, you can use this eating experience as an opportunity to learn something about your needs. You might say to yourself, *That salad was fine, but it felt like something was missing. It would have felt better to have a sandwich* (or some of the salad along with a sandwich, if you enjoyed the taste). *Good to know for next time!* Making that mind-body connection will help strengthen your ability to know what foods will satisfy you at a particular time.

How does this feel to you?

_____

_____

_____

_____

_____

I'll always get to eat again!

As you become an attuned eater, food becomes a source of nourishment and pleasure rather than angst and guilt. You no longer have to go for hours without eating because it's "not time to eat" according to your food plan. And when you give yourself a simple reminder that you can enjoy eating throughout the day, it may help you not feel the need to eat to a point of discomfort now.

To the extent that your circumstances prevent you from eating exactly when you're hungry, such as a work schedule with a specific lunch break, you can experiment with different patterns of feeding yourself that will keep you going throughout the day. The key is to adapt to real-life circumstances without restriction.

How does this feel to you?

_____

_____

_____

_____

_____

I can eat as much as I want. I'll do my best to pay attention to how my body feels.

Only _you_ get to decide how much you want to eat and how you want your body to feel when you're done. No one else knows what your body needs—not your partner, a parent, the chef at the restaurant, or us! By staying aware, without judgment, you'll develop a stronger sense of how much to eat to feel the way you want to feel.

How does this feel to you?

_____

_____

_____

_____

_____

I feel too full. I'll do my best to wait until I'm hungry again.

Just about everyone eats past fullness sometimes. But not everyone reacts in the same way. If you're in the diet mindset, you may find that as you keep eating to uncomfortable levels, you tell yourself to keep going because you've already broken through the restraints. Or you may punish yourself for your perceived transgression by undereating the next day. But by the evening, you are too hungry again and eat in a way that feels out of control. In either case, these reactions perpetuate the diet cycle.

Instead, consider responding from a place of compassion: *I'm uncomfortably full. It happens sometimes. I'll do my best to stay gentle with myself.* While this may sound contradictory, we suggest that even if you're not as hungry the next morning, you eat something to prevent a pattern of undereating during the day and making up for it at night.

How does this feel to you?

_____

_____

_____

_____

The Process of Learning Attuned Eating

When you're in the diet mindset, you're either "on" or "off" your plan. If you override your restrictions, you may eat in a way that feels chaotic until you impose control again. Then, you start over yet again and resume your previous restrictions—or try a new restrictive plan.

The process of learning attuned eating requires making a 180-degree turn. Here are some strategies to keep in mind as you embark on this journey.

Collect Attuned Eating Experiences

Imagine you have two baskets. One basket is for the times you eat that have nothing to do with physical hunger. Instead, you're turning to food in response to deprivation, habit, or emotional distress. Chances are that this basket is full right now.

The other basket is for the times that you practice attuned eating. Although this basket may not be very full right now, you can practice collecting attuned eating experiences. Each time you're hungry and eat something that satisfies you, place it in that basket. Just like putting money in the bank, it doesn't go away. You're likely to notice that these experiences feel good both physically and emotionally—and that's the incentive to keep moving in the direction of attuned eating.

To fill up your basket, use these prompts to note some recent attuned eating experiences:

When I was hungry, I ate _____.

Physically, it felt _____.

Emotionally, it felt _____.

The next time I was hungry, I ate _____.

Physically, it felt _____.

Emotionally, it felt _____.

Another time I was hungry, I ate _____.

Physically, it felt _____.

Emotionally, it felt _____.

When I was hungry again, I ate _____.

Physically, it felt _____.

Emotionally, it felt _____.

Watch this collection of attuned experiences grow over time!

As you collect attuned eating experiences, keep in mind that you may initially find yourself eating when hungry and stopping when full most of the time. While this will likely feel wonderful, you may be turning attuned eating into what is often called the *hunger/fullness diet*, where the new rules are "I can only eat when I'm hungry" and "I have to stop as soon as I'm full." Keep in mind that hunger and fullness are guideposts that are used to help you stay connected to your body. They're not meant to be used with rigidity. Instead, continue the process of collecting attuned eating experiences when you can.

Learning the process of attuned eating happens at a different pace for each person. If you only have one experience during the next week where you're hungry and eat something that satisfies you, that's terrific! If it happens more than once, that's terrific too.

For most people, it's also easier to figure out when to start eating than when to stop. That's okay! Over time, as you internalize the belief that food will always be available and won't be taken away by diet restrictions again, you will likely find that it feels safer to stop eating when you've had enough.

Reflect on Positive Eating Experiences

As you move in the direction of attuned eating, we can guarantee that you'll face challenges along the way. In the diet mindset, it's familiar to hear people say, "I've had a bad week" or "It's been a bad day" in reference to what they ate, and you may find yourself using similar phrases when you assess your attuned eating experiences.

In his book *Buddha's Brain*, neuroscientist Rick Hanson (2009) explains that our brains are like Velcro for the negative and Teflon for the positive. We tend to pay attention to negative events in our lives more so than positive ones. From an evolutionary perspective, this negativity bias makes sense. When our ancestors lived in the woods and heard a sound, they needed to think the worst—that it was a bear—and run. After all, if it was a bear and they didn't flee, you can imagine what would have happened. Our brains have become wired over time to expect the worst as a matter of survival. But that kind of thinking doesn't serve us if our experiences are not life-threatening.

Therefore, as you're in the process of collecting attuned eating experiences, it's important to notice not only your challenges, but your successes too. One client remembered a wonderful meal she had of grilled chicken kebabs, rice, veggies, and a slice of cake. Another client described the pleasure of eating his mother-in-law's delicious lasagna along with a salad and some bread. It's this awareness that allows you to collect attuned eating experiences in your basket. According to Rick Hanson, taking time to focus on these experiences by closing your eyes and holding them in your attention as you let them fill your mind and spread through your body, known as *taking in the good*, helps weave positive feelings into your brain and whole being.

When you're having a challenging time, take a moment to reflect, closing your eyes if that's comfortable for you, and use the following prompt: *I want to address some of the challenges I experienced this week. Before I do, let me think about whether any eating experience felt good. If so, I'll take a moment to hold the experience in my mind and recall how it felt in my body.*

Cultivate Compassion

As you collect attuned eating experiences, you'll find that there are plenty of times that eating doesn't go the way you wanted. Perhaps you eat to discomfort, eat something that doesn't feel good in your body, or start to eat when you're not at all hungry. This is to be expected! In the diet mindset, the default is to become upset with yourself. "I blew it," you might bemoan.

With attuned eating, there's nothing to "blow." Instead, it's about cultivating self-compassion to help you be curious about what happened without self-criticism. Self-compassion is about treating yourself with kindness and understanding in the face of difficulty or hard times, instead of judging or berating yourself. For many people, finding words of self-compassion can be difficult. If that's true for you, think about what you might say to a friend or child who is experiencing similar distress. Here are some phrases to help you get started:

- "I feel too full right now. That's going to happen sometimes as I learn how to listen to my body."

- "Sometimes I can't wait until I'm hungry to eat. I think something is bothering me and this is the best way I have to deal with it right now."

- "I didn't make the match. I think I'm still judging what I eat and not letting myself get what I really want. I know it's going to take time to undo years of the diet mindset."

Now it's your turn! In the spaces provided, write some compassionate statements. You might return to this page and add more as you think of them further down the road.

_____

_____

_____

_____

_____

_____

_____

_____

_____

Come back to these statements as often as you need to shift the way you talk to yourself about food.

Common Challenges in the Process of Learning Attuned Eating

The basic concept of attuned eating is simple: Eat in response to hunger and stop in response to satiation, most of the time. But there's nothing easy about it! All kinds of factors can interfere with this ability, and this is especially true for people who've been caught in the diet cycle. You've been taught that your body can't be trusted and that you therefore should disconnect from it.

While people caught in the diet cycle have a lot in common, it is also true that each person's journey is unique. The challenges _you_ confront along the way are part of the process, not an indication that you're doing something wrong. As you approach these challenges with compassion and curiosity, you can develop new strategies to support your needs.

Here are some common challenges that arise for people as they move in the direction of attuned eating. Think about which ones you can relate to.

Judgment

It takes time to let go of the "good/bad" thinking you've internalized about food, and that judgment can get in the way of truly giving yourself permission to eat what you're hungry for. If you have trouble choosing something satisfying to eat, ask yourself whether at some level you aren't allowing yourself to eat the food you really want to. Remind yourself that all foods fit.

Not Having Food Available

In order to eat foods that will satisfy you, it's important to have them available to the extent you can given your budget. Make sure to keep foods in your home that you find nourishing and pleasurable—and don't forget to take that food bag with you when you're out of the house so you can make sure you're not in a situation where you become ravenous.

Habitual Patterns

If you find that you automatically eat out of habit in certain situations, see if you can become curious about the pattern. Does it serve you in some way? Is it a pattern you'd like to change? For example, if you automatically eat popcorn when you go to a movie theater, does that habit enhance your moviegoing experience? If the answer is yes, but you also notice you become overly full in a way that feels uncomfortable to you, how can you "arrange" your hunger so that eating the popcorn feels better in your body?

Psychological Factors

Even as you experiment with strategies to support attuned eating, you may find that certain psychological issues impact your process. For example, perhaps you grew up in a family where you weren't allowed to express your needs, so you got good at pushing them down to keep yourself safe. As a result, noticing your hunger, which is a need, feels scary.

Perhaps you grew up in a family where your weight was a constant focus, and you worry that if you don't keep pursuing weight loss, you'll be rejected by your family. Perhaps you are overwhelmed by the tasks of life. Just the thought of preparing food for yourself, let alone bringing along a food bag, feels impossible. You long for the day that someone else takes care of you.

If barriers such as these get in the way of attuned eating, then it's important to decide how to address them. You might remind yourself that you're no longer in a situation where you're punished for your needs. You might realize that your family also bought into diet culture and reject their beliefs about your need to pursue weight loss. You might explore how to integrate self-care into your life, to the degree possible. But if you find that you cannot address these challenges on your own, there are knowledgeable professionals who can support you in this process.

Your Unique Challenges

Use this space to name some of the challenges you've become aware of when it comes to attuned eating. For each challenge, brainstorm some concrete strategies you've learned about in this chapter that might help, such as keeping a food bag, reminding yourself that all foods are permissible, cultivating compassion, and so on. If concrete strategies don't work, you may need to dig deeper. If you feel stuck, you may want to get additional support from an anti-diet professional should this be accessible for you.

What are some of your challenges in practicing attuned eating?

_____

_____

_____

_____

_____

What are some strategies to help you work through these challenges?

_____

_____

_____

_____

_____

After you identify some strategies, put them into practice! How well did they work? Did you notice any additional barriers? If so, how might you address them?

_____

_____

_____

_____

_____

Relief and Grief

As you let go of the diet mindset, you may experience great relief. No longer do you need to count calories, fat grams, or carbs, or punish yourself for what you eat. At the same time, you may also experience loss. You've spent lots of time focused on diets and food plans in the pursuit of weight loss. You were promised that once you lost weight, you'd be more attractive, more successful, sexier, healthier, and happier. That's a lot to let go of.

In *The Diet Survivor's Handbook*, Judith and her co-author Ellen Frankel (Matz & Frankel, 2006) apply the stages of grief to the meaning of the end of diets. Spend some time thinking about where you are in the process.

- **Denial:** You wonder if you must truly give up on diets and the belief that you can permanently lose weight. You likely know someone who's been able to do that, so why can't you? Keep in mind that this person is a unicorn, and remember that more than 95 percent of people who diet for weight loss regain the weight. If you were going to be part of that small percentage, chances are you wouldn't be here!

- **Anger:** Perhaps you're angry that your sibling got the thinner genes in your family while you look more like your heavier parent or grandparent. Or as you learn about the physiology of dieting, you might notice anger toward a pediatrician who suggested food restriction at an early age, toward friends who keep making comments about weight, or toward a family member who pressures you to lose weight. Expressing anger toward diet culture can actually be a healing part of your journey.

- **Bargaining:** Even though an anti-diet approach makes sense to you, you might be tempted to diet "one more time" in the hope of losing weight and *then* implementing attuned eating. Unfortunately, that strategy is highly likely to fail because of the pitfalls of dieting.

- **Depression:** You're being asked to give up dieting behaviors and the fantasies of what life will be like for you once you lose weight. You may have organized much of your life around thinking about food and may even have developed friendships or a sense of belonging via weight-management groups. You've had the belief that "Once I lose weight, I'll be happy, successful, attractive, and healthy"—and that's a lot to give up too. If you're at a higher weight, you've likely experienced stigma or fat shaming, and trying to move out of a marginalized identity is another aspect of letting go of dieting that can feel hard to give up.

- **Acceptance:** You've reached the place where you accept the inherent failure of diets and let go of the pursuit of weight loss. You understand that dieting wreaks havoc on your well-being, and you're no longer willing to subject yourself to the physical and emotional harm that comes from dieting. You're open to taking care of yourself in the best way you can. You practice accepting yourself and others in their wholeness and live a life of increased freedom and authenticity.

These stages of loss are not always distinct, and you may find yourself experiencing two stages simultaneously or moving back and forth between stages.

Use this space to notice where you're at in your journey of relief and grief.

_____

_____

_____

_____

_____

_____

_____

_____

Attuned Eating Leads to Attuned Living

As you let go of the diet mindset and learn the steps of attuned eating, you may feel like you're learning a new language. We hope you're enjoying this new way of speaking to yourself about your relationship with food. You may also find that this language transfers to other areas of your life. After all, when you move in the direction of attuned eating, you learn the following:

- *I have needs* (hunger).

- *My needs are specific* (what I'm hungry for).

- *My needs can be filled* (satiation).

We often hear people use metaphors to describe how attuned eating has extended to situations in their life that aren't food related. For example, Stevie explained that her new role at work was "a perfect match," and Jonathan realized he was "hungry" for more social contact.

Shoshanna described an unmet need related to visits from her family that left her house a mess. Now that she felt more entitled to meet her needs, she was able to be specific in her request that they keep the family room uncluttered by storing their belongings in the bedrooms with the doors closed. As a result of this shift, she felt much more satisfied by their visit.

Daniel expressed that socializing had become too exhausting and that he was going to cancel all future plans because his body needed more rest. As he explored his all-or-nothing thinking, he compared it to his work with attuned eating. Just as he had realized that his body didn't want only fruits and vegetables, it also didn't want only sweets. He had come to understand that all foods fit. Likewise, there was room for both socializing and rest once he tuned into his body and paid more attention to his energy levels.

Use this space to write about how attuned eating has led you to attuned living. You may want to return to this activity after you've gathered more attuned eating experiences over time.

_____

_____

_____

_____

_____

_____

_____

_____

_____

_____

We've given you a lot of information in this chapter, and it will take time to unlearn the diet mindset as you integrate the attuned eating framework. A helpful way to check in with yourself is through a timed-writing exercise. Use the space below or grab a blank piece of paper, choose any of the following prompts, and set your alarm to spend three to five minutes writing your response without censoring yourself. Don't worry about spelling or grammar—just let the words flow! Afterward, reflect on your response and see if it can help to guide you on your journey to make peace with food.

- When I think about letting go of dieting behaviors, I . . .

- The most exciting aspect of attuned eating is . . .

- The biggest challenge to becoming an attuned eater is . . .

- The next step for me in using this framework is . . .

_____

_____

_____

_____

_____

_____

_____

_____

_____

_____

_____

_____

_____

_____

_____

_____

_____

_____

_____

_____

Clinician's Corner

In this chapter, we explored skills and strategies to help people move in the direction of attuned eating. Take a pause and check in with yourself to see where you're at when it comes to working with clients in this arena. We've adapted the last activity of this chapter for that purpose. You can respond to any or all of the following prompts:

- When I think about letting go of dieting behaviors, I . . .

- When my clients think about letting go of dieting behaviors, they . . .

- The most exciting aspect of using attuned eating in my clinical work is . . .

- The biggest challenge to using attuned eating in my clinical work is . . .

- The next step for me in using this framework in my clinical work is . . .

_____

_____

_____

_____

_____

_____

_____

_____

_____

_____

_____

_____

_____

_____

_____

_____

Based on your responses, you can consider your next steps:

- If you already embrace attuned eating in your own life, you're likely comfortable teaching the skills in this chapter and exploring any challenges that arise with your clients.

- If you are new to the anti-diet approach and it rings true to you, you're in a strong place to support your clients on their journeys. You may wish to seek some additional training, consultation, or supervision to enhance your understanding of this framework. If you support an anti-diet approach but don't want to develop more of the skills to focus on eating and body concerns with your clients, consider referring them to a non-diet group, an intuitive eating course, or even another clinician who can collaborate with you and your client to offer counseling related to this topic.

- If you are on the fence with this approach or don't believe it could possibly work, it's important to provide your clients with other options to heal their relationship with food. If your client is learning about attuned or intuitive eating in another arena, please do your best to support their journey by listening to their experiences and refraining from making judgments about food and body size.

Most of the clinicians we know (including ourselves!) promoted dieting behaviors in some way in their clinical work before shifting to an anti-diet approach. In addition to keeping up to date on the research related to diet failure and the benefits of attuned eating, listening to the lived experiences of clients is a powerful means of learning. As you witness the relief and freedom clients discover as they practice attuned eating, you're likely to find great satisfaction in your role as an anti-diet clinician. This holds true even if you're in the process of making peace with food for yourself.

CHAPTER 4

Emotional Eating

The act of eating, in and of itself, is an emotional experience. It can offer feelings of satisfaction and pleasure. It can help you feel connected to your family, friends, and culture. Food is part of most celebrations, ranging from holidays to weddings to religious events. It's also present in times of loss at funerals or memorials. There's nothing inherently wrong with emotional eating!

At the same time, many people rely on food as their primary way to manage distress. If that describes you, this chapter will help you learn new ways to talk to yourself about food and cultivate strategies that can help you attend to your emotions without the further distress that can come from eating to discomfort or bingeing. As we explore these options, keep in mind the following:

- Even if you believe you're an emotional eater, it's extremely important to make sure that you've ended the deprivation that comes from food restrictions and that you're eating enough.

- You're not "bad" for turning to food in times of distress. Even as you learn other possible ways to cope, using food for comfort at times remains an option.

- As much as you may want to change emotional eating, be patient! The more attuned eating experiences you collect, the stronger the position you'll be in to address your emotional needs.

To help you begin to understand the role that emotional eating plays in your life, take a moment to think about the feelings that may lead you to turn to food, and jot them down here.

_____

_____

_____

_____

_____

_____

Just about any feeling can be at the core of your need to turn to food. You may be aware of the feeling. Or you may find yourself going to food but be unsure why you feel compelled to eat. Remember, if you're still restricting at any level, this can explain why you're turning to food.

Even though it may seem that the emotion is the reason you turn to food, it's not the feeling itself that causes you to eat. Rather, it's that you're having trouble *tolerating* the feeling at a particular moment. Think of it as an issue of emotion regulation. We all need ways to get through times of distress. Sometimes we find ways to comfort, calm, or soothe ourselves that help us tolerate a difficult time. Or we may feel too overwhelmed by what's happening and need to distract ourselves for the time being. When a feeling is so intense or unacceptable that it becomes intolerable, numbing can be a strategy to survive.

When you are having trouble tolerating your feelings, describe what the food does to help you at these times. Place a check mark next to the ones that resonate for you and add any other functions that food serves for you:

Soothes

Distracts

Comforts

Calms

Numbs

Other: _____

How you make your way through distress has a lot to do with what you've experienced throughout your life. If you've grown up with the experience of being seen and heard much of the time, you're more likely to be able to self-soothe in times of distress and to develop relationships that support you in managing the difficult times that are part of being human. But if you've grown up with the experience of being ignored, criticized, verbally abused, or physically abused, these skills may be less accessible to you.

In the next chapter, we'll focus more on trauma as it relates to emotional eating and BED. For now, let's explore why the use of food to manage emotions is so common and how the process of using food to cope actually works.

We've heard many people say that the emotional eating they engage in is an act of self-sabotage, but we see it differently. Trying to attend to your needs by regulating your emotions in some way is a positive action. Food is the first way we're soothed when we're born. When a baby cries, they're offered the breast or bottle. That early feeling of being cared for via food is wired into our psyche, so it makes sense that when you feel distress, food becomes your go-to. Not to mention that it's often available. Finding self-compassion for your need to turn to food is a great first step.

At the same time, we understand that ultimately, it's helpful to learn how to address feelings without using food so that you no longer experience the physical and emotional discomfort that can result from emotional and binge eating. You will also be in a stronger position to deal more effectively with the challenges you face.

Translating Feelings into the Language of Food and Weight

When it comes to emotional eating, most people think it goes like this:

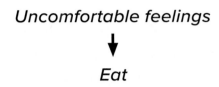

But it often happens more like this:

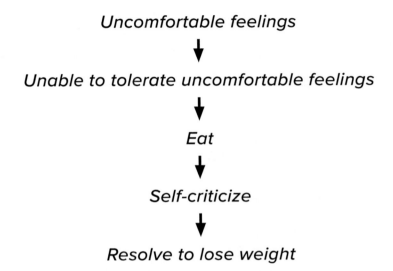

This common pattern leads you to focus on the wrong issue: losing weight. After all, resolving to lose weight won't help you solve whatever is really bothering you. Not to mention that the pursuit of weight loss is a setup because we know that restriction triggers rebound eating.

For example, Trisha found herself eating out of emotional distress after her kids finally went to sleep. She had eaten plenty for dinner and enjoyed a snack with her children before bedtime, so she knew she wasn't hungry. But she felt burdened by all of the responsibilities that fell to her as a single, working mom. As she ate popcorn and became increasingly physically uncomfortable, she berated herself. "I just keep getting bigger and bigger," she thought. "I have no self-control, and I need to lose weight. I'm going to go back to my diet on Monday." While Trisha resolved to lose weight, she continued to eat.

Trisha's thought process, which is typical for people who describe themselves as emotional eaters, was keeping her stuck. Let's take a closer look at what happened:

- Trisha was feeling burdened and resentful. It's understandable that she felt that way.

- Once her kids were asleep, Trisha was more aware of her feelings and tried to manage them the best way she could in that moment by turning to food.

- When she told herself that she needed to stop eating so she could lose weight, she translated the language of feelings to the language of food and weight. She felt burdened by her role as a single mom—but losing weight would not resolve that feeling.

- As she continued to criticize herself, she became more anxious and ashamed and kept using food to soothe herself.

- Trisha's promise to lose weight meant that the foods she enjoyed were going to be taken away again. This belief led her to eat even more popcorn that night because the typical response to impending deprivation is to think, *I better get more of it while I can.*

Does this pattern seem familiar to you? Use this space to write down any reflections about this pattern that you experience.

_____

_____

_____

_____

_____

_____

_____

_____

_____

The Role of Self-Compassion

The antidote to this pattern of emotional eating is self-compassion. In chapter 3, we talked about how to practice the skill of self-compassion when it comes to learning attuned eating. Here are some more ways that you can apply self-compassion to emotional eating, if it exists for you.

When you first start to let go of the diet mindset and move toward attuned eating, you may not be sure if you are reaching for food because of deprivation or as an attempt at emotion regulation. At this point, a simple phrase can help you speak kindly to yourself: *I'm reaching for food and I'm not hungry. I may be responding to deprivation, or there might be something bothering me, and this is the best way I have to take care of myself right now.*

The act of ending self-criticism and replacing it with self-compassion can actually reduce the amount of time you spend feeling out of control with food. Remember, all of that self-criticism just makes you more anxious and ashamed.

As you collect more attuned eating experiences, you're likely to feel calmer on the inside. You're building a new, reliable structure to guide you in deciding when, what, and how much to eat. You're ending deprivation-driven eating so that you're in a stronger position to dig deeper into emotional eating. Here's a phrase that can help you begin to explore the emotional aspects of eating: *I'm reaching for food and I'm not hungry. I wonder if there are feelings or thoughts I need to attend to?*

In the past, your reach for food blocked your access to what was really bothering you. As you build self-compassion and let go of self-criticism, you can begin to name the underlying feelings at the root of your emotional eating. For some people, this comes easily, while for others it's a new or challenging skill. Just about any feeling can lead you to turn to food, including sadness, anger, loneliness, boredom, and even happiness.

The following emotions wheel can help you identify your feelings. You may want to copy this chart and keep it in a handy spot to access when needed. You might find that being able to identify your feelings is calming in and of itself. Sometimes, though, identifying feelings can be unfamiliar or even stressful. With practice and support, you will find that feelings become easier to tolerate.

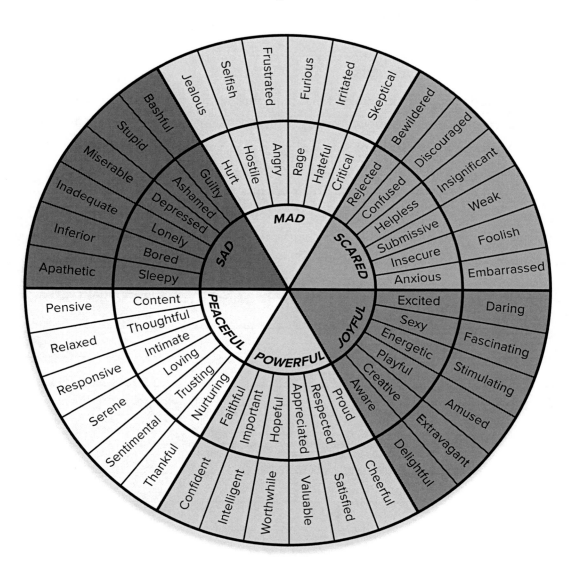

What Are You *Really* Hungry For? Cultivating New Strategies for Emotion Regulation

As you begin to identify feelings connected to your emotional eating, you can start to better understand why you are turning to food. When you notice yourself reaching for food and recognize it as an attempt to cope with emotions, you're learning to identify your feelings and needs in real time.

Go back to our checklist at the start of this chapter regarding the function of food and ask yourself what you need in that moment. Do you need to calm, comfort, soothe, distract, or numb yourself? If so, are there ways you can do that that don't involve food? For example, you might:

- Calm yourself by lighting a candle

- Comfort yourself by seeking connection with a friend

- Soothe yourself by being in nature

- Distract yourself by watching a movie

- Numb yourself by going to sleep

These are all emotion regulation strategies that may provide you with what you need in this moment. They are *not* strategies for controlling your eating. This is an important difference. Chances are that, at some point, you learned ways to control your eating via diet culture. For example, you may have been told to go for a walk, take a bath, or call a friend in order to avoid eating. As you make peace with food, remember that it's no longer about control. When you use control, the likely outcome is that you will eventually feel out of control. Instead, you're slowing down to ask yourself what strategies can help you manage and tolerate emotional distress. Remember, the food is still available if needed. You can always try other coping strategies in addition to eating.

Make a list of strategies that are currently available to help you cope with your emotions.

_____

_____

_____

_____

_____

_____

_____

_____

_____

Make a list of strategies that are not currently available but that you would like to cultivate to help you cope with your emotions. (Examples include learning a new hobby such as knitting, starting a journal, or learning a mindfulness practice.)

_____

_____

_____

_____

_____

_____

_____

_____

_____

The next time you find yourself reaching for food to manage an uncomfortable feeling, ask yourself what else you might be hungry for, in addition to food. For example, are you bored and hungry for stimulation? Are you lonely and hungry for connection? Once you identify the need, brainstorm a list of ways you might respond.

I'm hungry for: _____

Another way I can meet that need is: _____

_____

_____

_____

If you find that you're not able to respond to your feelings and meet your needs, remember the following:

- Food is always an option to deal with emotional distress.

- It takes time to cultivate new ways of coping.

- There are likely good reasons that you still use food as a source of comfort. Chapter 5 will give you a deeper understanding of why that may be and how you can further address these dynamics.

There are no rules for how you'll work your way through the emotional aspects of your eating. The journey looks different for each person. Just remember these steps to help you move through this process:

1. Ask yourself: *I'm reaching for food. Am I hungry?* If the answer is yes, or if it's the time you would typically eat, it's important to eat even if there's an emotional aspect to your reach for food.

2. If you're not hungry, try to be curious about what you're thinking or feeling that needs your attention. Even if you decide to go ahead and eat, you can reflect on how you might be using food to cope.

3. Making peace with food is never about control. Instead, give yourself permission to eat without criticism. Speak to yourself with compassion, remembering that this is the best way you have to take care of yourself right now.

Common Themes Behind Emotional Eating

As you work to build your coping skills, you may notice some common themes that lead you to reach for food. For each theme here, note if it applies to you and, if so, think of a time when it occurred. These patterns can become ingrained and take time to unlearn. With compassion, ask yourself if there's a next step you can take to move in the direction of coping with your emotions.

Setting Boundaries

Your boundaries are important. If you overextend yourself with family, friends, or work, you may not have adequate time to meet your own needs. Food becomes a way to get something for yourself.

> Andrew was the primary caretaker of his aging mother. As her needs for care increased, he became exhausted and unable to spend time with friends. He found himself eating to discomfort before bed as he tried to get something for himself before the day ended. Andrew eventually realized he needed to set some boundaries about what he could provide. He talked with his siblings, who agreed to help pay for a caregiver who could relieve Andrew of some of his responsibilities.

How might this theme apply to you, and what next step could you take to overcome this pattern?

_____

_____

_____

_____

_____

_____

Holding Two Feelings

You may find that it's difficult to hold two opposing feelings at once or that certain feelings are unacceptable to you. Eating becomes a means to push away an uncomfortable feeling.

> Jane felt relieved to have her twenty-something son home during the pandemic because it was safer for him. She also felt resentful that he was back home after she and her partner had adjusted to being empty nesters and enjoyed the freedom that came with this stage of life. Jane felt guilty that she resented her son's presence and turned to food to push away her resentment. As Jane learned that it's important and possible to hold both sets of feelings—she can feel relief that her son is home safe and resentment that he's always around at the same time—she could let go of the guilt and no longer needed to use food to regulate her emotions.

How might this theme apply to you, and what next step could you take to overcome this pattern?

_____

_____

_____

_____

_____

Rest and Replenishment

You may believe that taking time to slow down and rest is "doing nothing" and that you have to be productive. Turning to food can be a way to put off a task or chore that you believe you "should" do but don't have the energy for at a particular time.

> Shawn grew up with the message that sitting down when there were chores to be done was a sign of laziness. They often found themselves reaching for food to postpone paying the bills or doing the laundry. After all, at least eating was doing something! Shawn had to reflect on their own values to discover that their body needed rest at times, and this was a positive behavior. Reading a book, watching a TV show, or just sitting in their favorite comfy chair became a way to rest and replenish. They also realized that their concern (i.e., that they wouldn't want to do anything once they sat still) was unfounded and that their energy level was actually better overall when they tuned into their need for downtime.

How might this theme apply to you, and what next step could you take to overcome this pattern?

_____

_____

_____

_____

_____

_____

Perfectionism

If you're an all-or-nothing thinker, you may pressure yourself to get everything just right. One misstep and you believe you're a failure. This mindset creates anxiety and shame, and food can be a way to manage your distress.

> Nina was a high achiever who was admired for participating in numerous organizations on her college campus. But to keep up with her internal standards of success, she was depleted. She rarely slept more than five hours per night, and if she didn't get a perfect score on a test, or if she made a mistake in her volunteer roles, she felt devastated. Food was a way to comfort herself, and this compounded her distress. She tried to follow diet rules in an attempt to meet the cultural ideal of thinness, and when she broke through those restraints, she became increasingly anxious because she was used to doing things "perfectly." As Nina sought counseling to understand her out-of-control eating, she gradually understood the concept of being "good enough." Nina moved in the direction of attuned eating and worked on letting go of phrases such as "I must" and "I should" and accepting that everyone has strengths and weaknesses. She discovered that living in the gray helped to decrease her anxiety.

How might this theme apply to you, and what next step could you take to overcome this pattern?

_____

_____

_____

_____

_____

_____

Self-Care

It's important to practice self-care behaviors that support your physical, emotional, and spiritual needs to the extent possible given your circumstances. But food can sometimes become a substitute for these needs, such as when you use food to try to stay awake when your body needs sleep.

As a teen, Ella's parents told her that keeping her weight down was evidence of good self-care. As Ella focused on weight loss, she became stuck in the diet cycle. Paradoxically, food became a way to soothe her sense of failure about her body size based on the pressures from her family and diet culture. As Ella thought about what physical and emotional well-being meant to her, she realized that she needed to reject the diet mindset and start eating more. She also discovered that she truly enjoyed movement, such as dancing or walking, and that she needed to stop surfing the internet by 10:00 p.m. so she could get an adequate amount of sleep. As Ella implemented these behaviors, her mind felt clearer, and her physical energy level felt better. She continued to work on body acceptance and rejecting the messages she received about weight as self-care.

How might this theme apply to you, and what next step could you take to overcome this pattern?

_____

_____

_____

_____

_____

Regulating Your Nervous System: From Anxious to Calm

When you experience stress, your sympathetic nervous system becomes activated, triggering your body's fight-or-flight response and initiating the release of stress hormones, such as adrenaline and cortisol, into the bloodstream. This is a normal response to stressful situations, such as when you're speaking in front of an audience or going to a job interview. It's also necessary if you're in true danger and need to protect yourself from the threat at hand by running away or fighting back. But if your sympathetic nervous system is activated day in and day out, it can negatively affect your physical and mental health.

Since food is a coping mechanism that people often use to alleviate stress, learning how to calm your body and quiet your mind in other ways is important to help you shift your relationship with food. Food can't meet every need, so you need to discover other ways to calm your nervous system. In this section, we'll introduce two practices that can help you feel more grounded and present. Both of these practices activate the parasympathetic nervous system, which promotes rest and relaxation through the release of oxytocin, known as the calming hormone. Since you can't be anxious and calm at the same time, these practices can help alleviate stress.

Mindfulness Practices

As we discussed in chapter 3, mindfulness is about bringing your awareness to the present moment, without judgment. Mindfulness has become increasingly popular in our culture, with endless ways to learn and apply this practice. Some people prefer engaging in mindfulness practices they can do on their own, while others enjoy doing guided meditations. There are multiple paths to cultivating mindfulness, whether you prefer finding a teacher, searching the internet, or using an app. It may take time to find a practice that's right for you, or you may find that mindfulness is uncomfortable for you at this time. That's okay too.

Here's a simple mindfulness practice that involves diaphragmatic breathing. You can try it for a couple of minutes, five minutes, ten minutes, or however long serves you:

Diaphragmatic Breathing

To begin, find a comfortable place to sit, placing one hand on your chest and the other hand on your diaphragm, if that feels okay for you. Close your eyes and begin breathing through your nostrils so that the inhale is the same length as the exhale. See if you can keep your upper hand relatively still while your lower hand moves with each breath. As you breathe, you may find that your mind wanders to other thoughts, worries, or plans. That's okay! Whenever you notice your mind wandering, see if you can let go of your thoughts and come back to the breath, repeating as often as needed.

When you are done, describe what you experienced in a word or two: _____

_____

If you found this practice brought you a sense of peace, calm, or restfulness, consider repeating as desired. Keep in mind that engaging in regular practice helps build the capacity for mindfulness so that it's more accessible to you during times of stress.

Visualization Practices

Another technique to calm your nervous system is to practice visualization by taking yourself to a relaxed and peaceful place in your mind. When you feel uncomfortable feelings arise, see if this strategy can help you to get through the difficult moment. As with the diaphragmatic breathing exercise, you can try this practice for a couple of minutes, five minutes, ten minutes, or however long serves you.

Visualization

Close your eyes and take a nice, deep breath. Visualize yourself in a place where you feel calm and safe. It can be a place that you've been to or one that you imagine. Use your senses to notice what surrounds you: the sights, sounds, smells, and feel. You might also notice how your body feels as you let yourself enjoy this peaceful place. Spend some time here and remind yourself that you can always return to this calm and safe place. When you feel ready, slowly open your eyes.

When you are done, describe what you noticed in practicing this visualization: _____

_____

_____

If you find that these practices help you move through times of distress with more ease, that's terrific! You've added to the emotion regulation strategies you can use that don't solely involve reaching for food. If you find that these attempts to settle your mind and body are not accessible to you, it may be that experiences of trauma make it too uncomfortable to slow down and tune in. That's okay too. In the next chapter, we'll explore the connections between trauma and bingeing and support you in the journey toward healing.

Clinician's Corner

When you're seeing a new client with a history of chronic dieting, it can be helpful to ask them to ballpark what percentage of their eating is attuned eating. The answer will usually be low, ranging from zero up to somewhere around 30 percent. As your clients decrease their deprivation-driven eating, by definition, the percentage of their attuned eating experiences will increase. This puts them in a much stronger position to recognize when they are using food as a coping mechanism.

Additionally, as clients give themselves permission to eat all types of foods without judgment, they may find that food no longer does the same job of moving them away from difficult thoughts and feelings. After all, if clients allow themselves to eat chips when they're hungry for chips—and they no longer berate themselves for doing so—the chips may become less effective at moving them away from what is really bothering them. Judith often calls this moment with her clients "the good news and the bad news," explaining, "The good news is that you're no longer bingeing or eating to discomfort most of the time. The bad news is that you're left with painful feelings—but we know that's actually good news, too, because you can now work directly on these issues."

Your next steps depend on your scope of practice. If you're a therapist, this is the type of work you've been trained to do. If you're a clinician in another field, and you identify emotional issues that are beyond your scope, making a referral to a therapist who uses an anti-diet approach and who can collaborate with you is an important next step.

When clients turn to food with the awareness that they are not hungry, they may find it helpful to ask themselves, *What thoughts or feelings would I have if I didn't eat right now?* When this question is asked with compassion and curiosity after letting go of the diet mindset, clients often have more access to their emotional struggles that need exploration and healing. In the past, they turned to food and pushed away whatever was bothering them, often focusing on their eating behaviors and weight as "the problem." As they learn attuned eating, they decrease their anxiety around food and increase their ability to meet their needs. This puts them in a stronger position to become curious about the difficult emotions that still lead them to turn to food.

Therapists use all sorts of frameworks to help clients with all sorts of issues, and depending on your training, you're likely to apply the kind of approach you believe is best to help your client dig deeper into their emotional eating: psychodynamic therapy, cognitive behavioral therapy (CBT), acceptance and commitment therapy (ACT), dialectical behavior therapy (DBT)—the list goes on. We have found internal family systems (IFS) to be especially effective in treating emotional and binge eating because of its strengths-based perspective. No matter what type of framework you use, we believe it's important to help clients find compassion for how turning to food helps take care of the parts of them that are in distress, rather than feeling shame for their out-of-control eating. It's essential to help clients understand that they've done their very best to take care of themselves, even as they become curious about their emotional eating and search for other strategies to manage feelings.

It remains important to check in with clients about their attuned eating experiences to support them in keeping food as a source of nourishment and pleasure. Given the pressures of diet culture and the challenges of unlearning years (or even decades) of the diet mindset, it's understandable that they may run into challenges at times. Weaving together the concrete aspects of attuned eating with emotional exploration supports clients in the complex process of making peace with food.

CHAPTER 5

Binge Eating Disorder

Many people turn to food in times of distress. But sometimes, using food to deal with life becomes more frequent and extreme, and it may develop into binge eating disorder. This chapter will help you consider your eating patterns to determine whether you have BED and offer next steps to address the issue.

If you have BED (or suspect you might), you may feel discomfort, anxiety, or shame about your eating patterns while reading this chapter. One important thing to remember: People never choose BED, although some of the associated behaviors, like dieting, may start as a choice. BED is never about willpower. If you have an eating disorder, you have very good emotional and psychological reasons for it. BED often develops as a way to protect yourself when you have no other options.

As you consider your patterns with binge eating, try to offer compassion and curiosity, instead of judgment, to the parts of yourself that use food to soothe, escape, or distract. An important goal is to learn as much as possible about your relationship with food, and to do that, it needs to be safe for you to look closely at the role food plays in your life.

What Is Binge Eating Disorder?

As we discussed in the previous chapter, it's common for people to turn to food in times of distress. For some, the experience is short-lived, and the eating episodes are mostly conscious decisions. Picture eating a carton of ice cream after a breakup or eating a pizza in one sitting when you're worried about a work situation or a conflict with a friend. These are certainly potentially distressing events that may trigger the desire to soothe or distract yourself with food. But once the stressor is passed or resolved, your eating habits return to their previous patterns fairly quickly. Simply put, you are minimally affected by this bump in the eating road.

BED is fundamentally different and much more entrenched in a person's life than occasional emotional eating. A considerable part of a person's day might be organized around binge eating, and the binge episodes are more severe and frequent. Binge eating also typically begins earlier in life and is more complex to change. Additionally, people with BED feel a lack of control during a binge. The episodes feel impulsive and impossible to stop. People may even describe feeling "checked out" during a binge (clinically referred to as *dissociation*).

This lack of control is a hallmark of BED. Binge eating is something a person feels compelled to do, despite the significant shame that follows. The drive to binge overpowers the conviction not to, time and again. A client of Amy's talked about the urge being so powerful that she would be sitting on the sofa frantically eating food that she did not even taste while literally planning the next day's diet strategy: "I already feel bad about a binge before I even begin because I know I won't be able to stop it. It feels like a foregone conclusion before I take the first bite."

Because BED brings significant struggles with shame, people with the disorder, especially people in larger bodies, will typically work very hard to conceal this behavior. They may hide food in various locations, such as sneaking chips in their car or chocolate in the back of their desk drawer, and then eat "perfectly" in front of other people. As a result of such secrecy, binge eating is very isolating. For many, no one in their world knows about the behavior—or the emotional and cognitive turmoil that accompanies it. This leads to a vicious cycle where people socially isolate and increase their use of food to numb feelings of shame, only to feel even more shame.

People with BED often struggle with symptoms of depression or anxiety as well. Sometimes these symptoms are a result of binge eating, sometimes they're a cause, and sometimes it's both. Regardless, BED causes extreme distress, robbing people of time and energy and causing intense shame.

Does anyone in your world know about your binge eating?

_____

_____

Would it be helpful to get support? Who might be a good person to support you?

_____

_____

What would you like them to know?

_____

_____

_____

_____

The Symptoms

These are the official criteria for a BED diagnosis. Put a check mark by any statements that feel familiar to you:

Recurrent episodes of binge eating that occur at least once a week for three months

Eating a larger amount of food than would be considered "normal" in a short time frame

Feeling out of control and unable to stop the binge episode

Binge eating episodes are also associated with three or more of the following:

Eating until uncomfortably full

Eating large amounts of food when not physically hungry

Eating much more rapidly than normal

Eating alone out of embarrassment over the quantity eaten

Feeling disgusted, depressed, ashamed, or guilty after eating

In addition, here are some behaviors and thought patterns common to many people with BED. Put a check mark next to any statements that feel true for you:

My binge eating can feel frantic and out of control.

I often feel considerable shame or guilt when I binge.

My eating episodes often have a pattern (e.g., similar time of day, place, or types of foods eaten).

I eat in secret or hide food so I can binge on it later.

I think about binge eating throughout the day.

I feel "checked out" or emotionally numb when I'm binge eating.

I feel ambivalent about change. Part of me wants to stop binge eating and part of me is afraid to let it go.

While binge eating in BED is typically defined as eating a lot of food in a relatively short period of time, it can sometimes look more like grazing, taking place over many hours. People may still eat significantly more food than their body requires, but it happens throughout the day (or night) instead of in one discrete period of time.

People may also have periods when binge eating is less frequent or even stops, but then returns. The binge cycles characteristic of BED are less amenable to simple change techniques, like challenging negative thoughts or stopping dieting. If you have BED, letting go of the diet paradigm is critical, but it's usually not enough for long-term change. Typically, treatment with a trained professional is necessary.

In addition, while there is often the assumption that only people of higher weight can struggle with binge eating, BED impacts people of all body shapes and sizes. People with BED can be clinically considered "underweight" or be malnourished. In fact, food restriction is often part of developing BED. People at higher weights can have other types of eating disorders, too, or they may have no disordered eating at all. Keep in mind that the definition of BED does not mention weight, and recovery from BED is never about a number on the scale.

If you struggle with BED, you are certainly not alone. BED is three times more common than all other eating disorders combined and more prevalent than breast cancer, HIV, or schizophrenia. It is also by far the most common eating disorder among men, as 40 percent of people with BED identify as male (Hudson et al., 2007).

BED and ADHD

BED has a significant correlation with attention-deficit/hyperactivity disorder (ADHD). Up to 30 percent of people with BED also are on the ADHD spectrum (Geuijen et al., 2019). Difficulty with impulsivity is common to both BED and ADHD, as is difficulty dealing with big emotions. People with ADHD and BED may also struggle with other impulsive behaviors like shopping, gambling, and addiction. Relationships and work life can be significantly impacted by both disorders as well. For many, ADHD symptoms may be activated by certain childhood experiences or attachment patterns. If this is your experience, you may want to address these issues with a mental health professional. Working on your ADHD symptoms can be helpful in resolving co-occurring binge eating.

How Bingeing Helps

For many people with BED, there is a long history of turning to food to deal with emotions, stressors, and shame. As difficult as the experience of BED can be, often the prospect of stopping the behaviors can seem even more challenging. That's because binge eating creates a temporary disconnection from pain or fear. As one client put it, "Planning a binge gave me a safe harbor when I was afraid or lonely. It got me through my past, through my divorce, through a whole lot of pain I had no idea how to address."

In their book *Binge Eating Disorder*, Amy and her co-author Chevese Turner (Pershing & Turner, 2019) quote another client who described, "When I decide to binge, I'm free. There is nothing like it. I can feel my body relax and then kind of disappear. Then I see the evening ahead of me. Just me, the TV and the food, then sleep. A kind of sleep you can't get without bingeing. There won't be room for anything, or anyone, else. I won't think about all the things I'm going to screw up tomorrow, or who doesn't like me, or who is going to leave me" (p. 5).

There are a number of theories that attempt to explain, on a neurological level, why binge eating provides short-term relief when you are faced with a tremendous amount of anxiety, depression, or shame:

- Some studies suggest that when you consume foods high in sugar and fat, it temporarily enhances dopamine (the "feel-good" hormone) levels in the brain. This also lowers the production of stress hormones, like cortisol, in the short term (Rada et al., 2005).

- The enteric nervous system, which is a complex network of nerves that regulates stomach activity, may play a role as well. When you binge eat, it may reduce the stomach sensations associated with stress, like feeling sick to your stomach or feeling butterflies (Stanculete et al., 2021).

- During a binge episode, your prefrontal cortex (your "thinking brain") and your limbic system (your "emotional brain") are both less active because your body is focused on digestion. This, in turn, results in a numbing effect on emotional and cognitive awareness (Rada et al., 2005).

- Researchers have found increased levels of ghrelin (the "hunger hormone") among individuals with a history of early trauma, which may explain why they use food to soothe (Shin et al., 2023).

Use the space below to reflect on the ways binge eating may have helped you.

_____

_____

_____

_____

_____

_____

_____

Consider offering compassionate curiosity to the part of you that used eating a way to cope. Even though binge eating may feel destructive in many ways now, it might well have been profoundly helpful when it first developed.

Common Patterns

People with BED often have patterns in their binge eating behaviors. For example, you may binge on the same foods or types of foods, or have specific foods you turn to in response to different situations or moods. You may have specific places where you binge as well, such as in bed, on the couch, or in the car. Over time, these places may in and of themselves trigger the desire to eat.

In addition, most people with BED binge while engaging in another activity, such as watching television, surfing the internet, or reading. You may even have specific shows, websites, or books you turn to during a binge episode. It is rare for people to binge without distractions, as this quiets the small voice that is actually hoping to *stop* the behavior. Binge eating with distractions allows the experience of checking out of the world to be more complete. As one client put it, "I come home and turn on my binge shows before I have a chance to decide not to do it. I put on my loosest clothes, turn off the phone, and eat. I want salty then sweet, in that order, over and over. It's the same pattern, every time."

Use this space to write down any reflections about your patterns of binge eating. Include times of day, specific locations, and other activities associated with your binge eating. Notice how you feel exploring this information. Remember that you don't need to change any of these patterns until you feel ready to do so. This is just to help you be more aware of the patterns as they currently exist.

Trauma and BED

Although chronic dieting, food restriction, and body shame are all contributing factors to BED—with up to 70 percent of people with BED believing that dieting led to their binge eating—these factors, while powerful, are not the whole story. For most people with BED, traumatic experiences, especially those that occur in early life, are major contributing factors. In one study, 83 percent of patients with BED reported some form of childhood maltreatment (Westerberg & Waitz, 2013).

Traumatic experiences can take many different forms, as trauma is any experience or event that overwhelms your ability to cope. This can include growing up in an environment where you did not experience enough soothing touch or where your caregivers frequently displayed contempt or impatience in response to your emotions or needs. Your caregivers may have had traumatic experiences of their own, which taught you to be afraid of the world in response to their depression, anxiety, or shame.

Sometimes, the trauma you experienced may have been more severe. This can include being physically or sexually abused, growing up in poverty, being part of a stigmatized or oppressed group, and bullying (with weight-related bullying, in particular, often contributing to BED). These forms of trauma have a profound impact on how you experience the world.

No matter the form of trauma that you endured, the lack of control common in binge eating is often deeply driven by trauma. You are genetically and biochemically wired to find ways to cope with your environment. If you grew up in a world that was unsafe, chaotic, or dangerous, your body and mind learned how to compensate to allow you to survive. And, often, it compensated through behaviors like binge eating, which soothed overwhelming or confusing emotions.

If you are a trauma survivor, you might struggle with the following emotional symptoms, particularly in relationships. Check any symptoms that resonate with you:

Low self-esteem

Fear of trying new things or being in new situations

Difficulty identifying and describing emotions

Excessive worry about how you're perceived by others

Difficulty putting your own needs first

Difficulty maintaining relationships

Inability to deal with conflict in relationships (often due to a fear of rejection)

Difficulty setting boundaries or standing up for yourself

Pervasive sadness or hopelessness

Irritability or anger

Risky or potentially harmful behaviors (e.g., alcohol and drug use, reckless driving, overspending, missing medication doses)

Trouble concentrating

Difficulty trusting others

Struggles with intimacy

Pervasive feelings of isolation or loneliness

Mood swings ("big" emotions about "small" issues)

Panic or extreme fear

Inability to experience joy or spontaneity

You might also struggle with physical symptoms. (Be aware that unexplained physical symptoms may or may not have causes related to trauma, but possible connections to past experiences are important to explore). Put a check mark by any that ring true for you:

Muscle tension and chronic headaches

Shallow breathing

Exaggerated startle response

Flashbacks or intrusive images of the past

Unexplained chronic pain or fatigue

Hypervigilance

Insomnia or hypersomnia

Chronic gastrointestinal problems

If you experienced trauma early in life, parts of you may continue to view your current life through the lens of these past experiences. You may be frozen in the time of the trauma, leading you to interpret current events as similarly dangerous, even if they're unrelated to the events from your past. Your brain literally has a harder time realizing that the scary things that happened are in the *past*.

Binge eating is a very effective tool to cope with this sense of ongoing danger in the world because it helps you disconnect from your emotions and reactions. From this lens, bingeing is not a result of "pathology." It is an adaptive behavior, given the circumstances. The problem is that this also leads you to live disconnected from your body, with little sense of a physical anchor in the world. This disconnection is a very big contributor to binge eating. Healing from BED requires you to heal your relationship with your body and learn to feel safely connected to your needs and feelings.

What changes for you if you think of your binge eating as a way to cope with difficult or traumatic experiences?

_____

_____

_____

_____

_____

_____

POWR: A Process for Healing

People who recover from BED are able to develop a much more peaceful relationship with food and movement, increasingly based on good self-care. Binge eating may still happen sometimes, but it is less frequent and severe, and when it happens, they are better able to respond to themselves with compassion and curiosity.

One tool that can facilitate your healing is known as POWR, which is a strategy you can use when you feel the urge to binge. You may still decide to go to food, but this process can give you the space to have more clarity about what your needs might truly be in that moment, as well as space to consider other options. The steps of POWR are:

- **P**ause into presence

- **O**pen and allow

- **W**isely consider

- **R**espond with care

Let's explore each step. If any part of the POWR process feels too uncomfortable for you, make a note of the experience and stop for now. You can return to this process when you feel ready.

Pause into Presence

Usually, binge eating is all about checking out from your needs and sensations, not checking in. But checking in with yourself when you feel the drive to binge can help you learn more about what your real needs might be. Pausing into presence creates space for you to assess what's happening in the moment and determine what, if anything, you need to do to care for yourself. Here are the steps involved in this process:

1. Say to yourself, "I am having the urge to binge right now." Naming your experience in this way brings your prefrontal cortex (the "thinking brain") back online, helping you observe your experience from a slight distance. This helps create a little room from the sensations you may be feeling.

2. Remind yourself, "I am not in danger. I am safe, in the present."

3. Gently try a grounding exercise. (Two possibilities are included below.)

4. Say to yourself, "I can offer compassion to the part of me that wants to turn to food right now. I can be curious about what that part needs me to know. The food is there if I need it."

Tuning into your inner experience may be new for you and possibly uncomfortable or even frightening. If checking in feels scary for you, try to first remember a time when you felt deep compassion for someone who was struggling. Perhaps someone you love was faced with a significant loss. What did it feel like? How did your body experience this kindness and warmth toward another person? Can you offer that same energy to the parts of yourself that are afraid, just for now, as you try this exercise?

Square Breathing

This technique invites you to make a "square" with your breath. Notice what happens in your body with each step:

1. Breathe in to the count of four. Breathe in as deeply as possible.

2. Hold your breath for a count of four.

3. Slowly and evenly release your breath for a count of four.

4. Rest for a count of four before starting again.

5. Do this process four times.

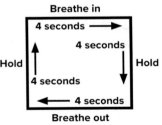

See My Hands

To begin, simply place your hands on your lap, resting them in whatever position feels most comfortable to you. Now, bring your attention to where your hands are touching your lap and where there are gaps. What is the difference in the sensations? What is the temperature of your hands? Is it constant throughout each hand? Do you notice any stress or pain in your hands? Do you notice any other physical sensations?

Now, notice how your hands appear, including your nails and knuckles. Where are they wrinkled? Or smooth? Do you see any color variation? As you finish, try to consider all the work your hands have done for you.

Open and Allow

This step of POWR is about noticing, with curiosity and without judgment, your experience in the moment. What sensations, emotions, or thoughts are you having right now? What is happening outside in your immediate environment? Consider the step of "open and allow" to be like watching a movie about your current experience. You are taking stock of your situation and identifying what you feel.

Name (aloud, if possible) your experience right now. Saying it out loud helps activate your prefrontal cortex, allowing you to step further into the present moment. List any sensations, emotions, or thoughts you are having without judgment. Just notice your current experience.

_____

_____

_____

_____

_____

_____

Wisely Consider

This step invites you to explore the beliefs that might be impacting how you're feeling in the moment. Often, these beliefs (called *schemas*) are formed in response to your experiences in childhood. For example, you might have learned that if you don't do something just right, you are a failure. Or you might have learned that people won't like you if you have needs of your own.

Your schemas may be hiding underneath the specifics of what is happening at the moment. For example, you may feel rejected or abandoned if someone cancels plans with you, even if they have a good reason to cancel and are a trusted friend. This, in turn, may lead you to believe that you're unlovable. This reaction is not about the present moment, but about times in early life when you felt abandoned by important caregivers. Schemas are typically global statements, all-or-nothing in nature, that feel very true—even though, at some level, you know they are distorted and extreme.

Here are some common schemas:

- I am fundamentally broken.

- I will be left alone if I am not perfect.

- I caused all the problems in my relationships.

- I can't let anyone see the "real" me, or I will be judged.

- I cannot trust my perceptions or my feelings.

To consider the schemas contributing to your urge to binge, ask yourself the following questions.

What belief, or schema, triggered your reaction?

_____

_____

Can you think of any childhood experience connected to this schema? How old were you when this experience occurred?

_____

_____

_____

_____

What are you hoping bingeing will change about this feeling or experience?

_____

_____

_____

_____

Respond with Care

This final step of POWR invites you to check in, identify what you really need right now, and then take any action you can to meet that need. Many people with BED did not receive the care and tenderness they needed in times of fear or pain. If this describes your experience, taking care of yourself now can feel revolutionary, and even scary or shameful. After all, you've learned to ignore your own needs for so long.

Good self-care is a big part of recovery, and with practice and time, it will become easier to respond to yourself with care without feeling the pull of fear or shame.

To determine what you need in this moment, look through this checklist and see if any of these needs might be present for you:

Support from others

Alone time

Reassurance

Space for your feelings

Time to grieve, celebrate, or explore a fear

The opportunity to cry, yell, write, run, or stretch

Time to be still and breathe

Sleep

Movement

Time spent outside in nature

The courage to allow something in or let something go

A break or time to play

Stronger (or looser) boundaries with someone

The strength to challenge something, accept something, or ask for something

The ability to just be present

Allow yourself to try to implement one or more of the actions you identified. See how it impacts your urge to binge. What changes do you notice? Was it difficult to allow yourself this good care?

_____

_____

_____

_____

_____

_____

Recovery from Binge Eating Disorder

Recovery from BED will take time, so it's important to approach your eating disorder with patience and compassion. Reconnecting with your body and working to heal your underlying wounds will not happen overnight, but with patience, you can learn to trust your body to tell you what it needs. Getting your life back from BED is the most important thing you may ever do. You are well worth the effort.

You might also benefit from working with a clinician or treatment team who is trained in the treatment of eating disorders from a strengths-based, weight-inclusive perspective, and who is well versed in treating trauma and other co-occurring concerns, such as ADHD.

Remember to offer compassion and gratitude to the part of you that reaches for food as a means of soothing or protection. This part of you has probably been doing this job for a long time and will need your help and guidance to change.

Clinician's Corner

Clients with BED will need to learn to identify and tolerate significant emotional and somatic experiences in order to heal. We have found that the best theoretical orientations are strengths-based, as they allow the client to be the expert in the room while also helping them feel supported in the therapeutic relationship. IFS therapy in particular is a powerful tool for helping clients access the safe space they need to explore their BED, heal trauma wounds, and work on changing old schemas. Eye movement desensitization and reprocessing (EMDR), somatic experiencing (SE), and other mindfulness-based approaches can be powerful additions to the IFS approach.

If you are working with clients with BED, we strongly recommend that you develop a working knowledge of the impact of traumatic experiences on neurodevelopment so you can share this information with your clients. When clients understand just how adaptive binge eating can be at the neurological level, they can release much of their shame about these behaviors. We have found that it is effective to use simple handouts or graphs explaining how the brain develops and encodes danger, such as those provided in Janina Fisher's (2022) *The Living Legacy of Trauma Flip Chart*. This knowledge can be depathologizing and empowering for many clients.

Additionally, it is crucial to empower your clients to survive in today's diet culture, where they may be retraumatized by messages related to body shaming and weight stigma. For some clients, it can be beneficial to find community or to participate in advocacy efforts to eradicate weight stigma.

No one clinician can know everything, so it's often helpful for clients to work with a treatment team when possible. This team might include a therapist, a dietitian trained in attuned eating and BED, a medical or psychiatric provider, and possibly a somatic practitioner. Additionally, pursuing training in areas such as neurodiversity and working with marginalized populations can help with diagnosis and treatment planning.

CHAPTER 6

Cultivating a Positive Body Image

We aren't born thinking about whether our bodies are good or bad. Think about a baby coming into this world. They love playing with their fingers and toes as they roll around in their crib. As they get older, you see toddlers and preschoolers running, jumping, skipping, and finding pleasure in the ways their bodies move. Young children aren't yet aware of the concepts of "thin" and "fat," and a parent's squishy tummy can be a source of comfort rather than a body part to be judged.

But early in life, children become exposed to messages that "fat is bad." These messages come from cartoons that portray fat characters as stupid or clumsy, the pediatrician who focuses on weight, and comments made by teachers or peers on the school playground. Even more insidious are explicit comments or implicit messages from parents and other family members conveying that a thin body is valued and that a fat body is shameful. Here's how some of these messages might sound:

- "Can you believe how much weight Aunt Eve gained?"
- "I can't have dessert. It's too fattening."
- "Are you sure you want another cookie? You know they have a lot of sugar."
- "My friend Meg lost so much weight and looks great. I want to find out what diet she's on."
- "No wonder your grandfather is sick. That's what happens when people are fat."
- "Your stomach sticks out in that shirt. You'd better be careful, or you'll gain more weight."
- "Nothing fits me. I don't like the way I look in these jeans."
- "I'll pay you for losing weight."
- "We only eat healthy foods in our house."

You get the idea. As a result of these kinds of messages, you may have come to believe that to be accepted and worthy, you need to lose weight or stay thin. You learn or experience that a larger body will be met with ridicule and rejection. In this way, our culture's negative attitudes toward body size, or weight stigma, are taught to you and internalized as your own beliefs. We refer to this as *internalized weight stigma*.

We understand that the people who transmitted these messages to you may have had your best interest at heart. They may have experienced the consequences of weight stigma themselves and truly believed that advising or pressuring you to be thin would protect you from the shame and harm they experienced.

They likely absorbed all the messages diet culture has to offer and believed that you would be happier and healthier in a thinner body.

They may not have realized the harm they were causing you physically and emotionally when they valued weight loss over your well-being. They didn't consider that body shame leads to disordered eating and eating disorders. They didn't know that getting caught in the diet cycle negatively affects health. They didn't realize that having a family accept you exactly as you are could help protect you, especially if you are in a larger body and subject to the weight stigma out in the world, and give you some resilience in the face of body shame and oppression.

It's not easy to unlearn the messages of diet culture. In this chapter, we'll give you some strategies to reject internalized weight stigma and move toward feeling more at home in your body. Keep in mind that this is hard work and takes place over time. Go at your own pace and take time to notice any moments where you feel discomfort.

At the same time, the stigma around weight and other marginalized identities that infiltrates our culture means that individual body image work will never be enough to solve the anti-fat bias that people are exposed to, especially if they're at a higher weight. Changing these attitudes and structures remains an important aspiration, and each of us can do our best to make sure we're not complicit in diet culture, and that we contribute to creating a more just and respectful world. We'll consider the bigger picture in chapter 9.

The History of Your Body

In chapter 1, we asked you to write your story about food, weight, and body image. Here are some questions to help you take a deeper dive into the source of your feelings toward your body. If you have the opportunity, these can be great conversation starters with other people in your life who are on the same journey or who are working with you in a clinical setting. Talking about body shame in a safe and compassionate space is healing and can even be empowering.

- When was the first time you felt shame about your body size?

- What were the explicit messages you received from others?

- What were the implicit messages you received from others?

- How did they develop their own beliefs about body size?

- If you could go back in time, what would you like to say to those people?

- Who benefits from your body shame? (Hint: Think diet, beauty, and wellness industries.)

- When you think about unlearning these internalized messages, what thoughts and feelings come up for you?

_____

_____

_____

_____

_____

_____

_____

_____

_____

_____

_____

_____

_____

_____

_____

_____

_____

_____

_____

_____

_____

As we offer strategies to unlearn these messages and cultivate a healthier body image, remember that your negative beliefs about your body are not your birthright. You learned these messages as the result of living in a culture that stigmatizes larger bodies and other marginalized identities, such as those associated with race, ethnicity, sexual orientation, gender, ability, and age.

No matter how much work you do to feel better about your body, if you're at a higher weight, the reality is that you'll continue to confront weight stigma from the people and systems you interact with, such as the medical profession and workplace. Ultimately, creating a culture that accepts and appreciates all body shapes and sizes is necessary to help you feel safe and respected.

Defining Body Image

People often talk about having a healthy or positive body image, but what does that really mean?

Take a moment to think of your own definition of body image and jot it down here.

_____

_____

_____

_____

Your body image isn't actually based on your body size. There are people at higher weights who experience positive feelings about their bodies, and there are people at the weight our culture considers "ideal" who experience negative feelings about their bodies. That's because body image stems from the *perception* someone has about their physical self and the thoughts and feelings they have about that perception. These thoughts and feelings may be negative, positive, or a combination of both.

Given the strength of internalized weight stigma, it's likely that you have negative thoughts about your body on a daily basis. These thoughts are so familiar that you may not even notice them, or you may think of them as "normal." But they affect how you feel about yourself and how your day will unfold.

Use this space to make a list of what you've said to yourself about your body in the past 24 hours.

_____

_____

_____

_____

_____

_____

_____

_____

When you read this list, how do you feel?

_____

_____

_____

_____

In their book *More Than a Body*, Lexie Kite and Lindsay Kite (2021) use the tagline, "Your body is an instrument, not an ornament." This simple sentiment is a helpful reminder as you move toward letting go of negative body thoughts.

Moving from Body Shame to Body Positivity

We know from neuroscience that what fires together, wires together, and you've succeeded in wiring these negative thoughts about your body into your daily life. You have these thoughts when you're choosing what to wear in the morning, looking in the mirror, or thinking about socializing with friends or family.

Because these thoughts have been wired into your brain, they've created a rut from which it can be difficult to break free. You can think of it like trying to back out of a snow-covered driveway. When you back your car out over the snow, it creates a deep groove that's hard to get out of unless you intentionally create a new path. Your task is to create a new path by changing the way you respond to these negative body thoughts—moving you from body shame toward more neutral or positive feelings toward your body.

When Judith and Amy (Matz & Pershing, 2020) created *The Body Positivity Card Deck*, they defined body positivity in the following terms:

> Body positivity means relating to your body with acceptance, appreciation and respect, rather than self-criticism, shame and body hatred.
>
> It doesn't mean loving your body 24/7. Instead, body positivity helps you unhook your body image from your value as a human being and supports you in cultivating practices that strengthen your physical, emotional, and spiritual wellbeing.
>
> Body positivity is for everybody: people of all sizes, shapes, colors, abilities, sexual orientations, gender identities, and ages.
>
> Body positivity includes rejecting cultural messages related to body shame and weight stigma and replacing them with messages that reflect acceptance and inclusiveness.

Here are some examples of body positive statements that foster greater acceptance, appreciation, and respect for one's body:

- **Acceptance**
  - "I look like my paternal grandmother. My thighs are thick just like hers."
  - "My body size is the result of my genetics, weight cycling, and other factors that are beyond my control."
  - "My body has changed as I've aged. I need to remember that bodies change through the life cycle."

- **Appreciation**
  - "My jiggly belly is the result of giving birth to my beautiful children. Isn't the human body amazing?"
  - "These are the arms that let me hug the people I love."
  - "My legs allow me to take walks in nature."

- **Respect**
  - "My body deserves to receive medical care that is free from fat shaming."
  - "I enjoy giving my body time to rest."
  - "I notice that my body likes to dance, so I'm going to make sure to play some fun music!"

In the following section, we offer various strategies to help you create greater body positivity and feel more at home in your body. These strategies will help you shift your attitude toward your body, make changes to your environment that support you, and ultimately integrate body acceptance into your daily life.

Strategies to Create an Attitude of Body Acceptance

Cultivate Self-Compassion

As we've discussed, learning to let go of diet culture can feel like learning a new language. When it comes to body acceptance, self-compassion is key. You're moving from the critical language of body shame to the language of kindness, compassion, and curiosity.

According to self-compassion expert Kristin Neff (2003), there are three components of self-compassion:

- **Self-kindness:** Talk to yourself with the same kindness and understanding that you would extend to a close friend or child.

- **Common humanity:** No matter what you're going through, remember that you are not alone. We're all connected in this world, and the nature of the human condition is that we all have struggles.

- **Mindfulness:** Instead of staying stuck in your feelings, observe them from the stance of an open, curious, nonjudgmental observer. Then think about one step you can take to care for yourself.

For example, Brenda, a college student, was heading home for spring break. She'd been working on attuned eating since the start of the semester, and her bingeing had significantly decreased. As she thought about being with her family, she also thought about the way they focused on weight and how shaming that felt to her. Here is how she applied the components of self-compassion to help her navigate the situation:

- **Self-kindness:** "I'm doing the best I can to heal my relationship with food. I know that this is the right path for me."

- **Common humanity:** "Lots of people have a hard time going to visit their families after living independently. I know that many families focus on weight loss."
- **Mindfulness:** "I'm feeling anxious and fearful of the comments I might hear from my parents since I haven't lost any weight."

From that place of self-compassion, she was able to brainstorm the following ways to take care of herself:

- "I will let them know ahead of time that I'm no longer dieting or focused on weight."
- "If they bring it up in conversation, I will change the subject."
- "If they won't let it go, I will go to my room or take a walk."
- "I will ask my friend Aron if he can be available if I need some support through text or a phone call."

The combination of setting boundaries and eliciting support helped Brenda navigate her visit home without the usual shame she felt about her weight. Brenda also gave herself permission to make alternative plans in the future if her family wouldn't respect her request.

To get into the habit of using self-compassion to create greater body acceptance, think of a situation, real or imagined, that would make you feel discomfort when it comes to the topic of weight. In the past, you may have joined in and agreed with the messages of diet culture. Instead, use self-compassion to think through how you can navigate these challenges in a way that leaves you feeling grounded, respected, or whole.

Situation: _____

_____

Self-kindness: _____

_____

Common humanity: _____

_____

Mindfulness: _____

_____

A next action I can take is: _____

_____

We also want to note that beyond body size and shape, there may be other factors that get in the way of feeling at home in your body, such as gender identity, physical ability, or chronic pain. To the extent that you don't feel at home in your body because of these factors, can you notice what your body is telling you it needs? Is there a way for you to offer your body compassion? For example, if you experience chronic pain, can you offer tenderness to those parts of your body?

Make a list of any factors that affect the way you feel about your body size and shape. For each factor, try to develop a compassionate response.

Factor	Compassionate Response

Mindful Awareness

Cultivating a positive body image doesn't require you to always feel positive about your body. Rather, you can shift your attitude by noticing the negative thoughts that pop up automatically without letting these thoughts take over. Notice the way you're feeling about your body right now. If you're having negative body thoughts, think of them as leaves floating on a stream, and allow them to pass by (rather than believing the thoughts and letting them move you back to the diet mindset). When a negative thought pops up, try to imagine placing it on a leaf and watching it float downstream. Repeated practice of this exercise can help you rewire your brain to let go of the automatic negative body thoughts.

The Computer Exercise

As you practice letting go of negative body thoughts, the next step is to replace them with new thoughts that convey body acceptance, appreciation, and respect.

To do so, close your eyes, if you feel comfortable doing so, and take a couple of deep breaths. Think of a recent negative thought you've had about your body, or one that comes up often for you, and imagine typing that thought on a computer. Now imaging pushing the delete button and watching that thought disappear! Try to replace that negative thought with a more compassionate statement that shows acceptance, appreciation, or respect. If you're having difficulty coming up with a thought, imagine that a dear friend were saying negative things about their body. How might you respond to them in a compassionate way? Now imagine typing that thought on your computer so you can see it on your screen. When you're ready, open your eyes.

Were you able to find a more compassionate way to talk to yourself? Many people find it challenging—and that's not surprising, given the judgmental way bodies are talked about in diet culture. Here are a few examples to help you reframe negative thoughts into a more compassionate correction:

Negative Thought	Compassionate Correction
"My body is in pain because of my weight."	"It's hard to be in pain. I'm doing the best I can to manage it."
"My stomach is gross."	"My stomach allows me to digest my food and feel satiated."
"I have to wear long sleeves in the summer to cover up my arms."	"My body deserves to feel cool and comfortable when it's warm outside."

While these new statements may feel awkward to you at first, repeated practice helps wire in more compassionate ways to speak to yourself about your body. You're learning a new language!

10 Tips to Help Your Child Develop a Positive Body Image

1. Avoid diet talk and dieting behavior in front of your child (and altogether, if possible!).

2. Avoid commenting negatively on other people's body weight, shape, or size, *as well as your own*, in front of your child (and again, ideally altogether).

3. Refrain from criticizing your child's weight or appearance.

4. Do not categorize foods as "good" and "bad."

5. Feed your child in ways that feel good to them, not based on body size.

6. Compliment your child on positive behaviors and characteristics, rather than focusing on body size and appearance.

7. Encourage physical activity for enjoyment and well-being, rather than weight control.

8. Promote a peaceful relationship with food. This includes honoring cues for hunger and fullness, providing a wide variety of all types of food, and sharing family meals when possible.

9. Support self-care behaviors, such as getting enough sleep, maintaining good grooming habits, and developing creative hobbies and interests, rather than focusing on weight loss.

10. Teach your child that people naturally come in different shapes and sizes and that everyone deserves to be treated with respect.

Strategies to Create an Environment of Body Acceptance

As you try to make changes from the inside out about the way you talk to yourself about your body, it can help to make changes in your environment that also support you. The following are some suggestions to get you started. Keep in mind that these are guidelines that have the potential to strengthen your body image. They're not meant to be new rules, so choose what is useful to you.

What's in Your Closet?

It's typical for people who are chronic dieters to have multiple sizes of clothes in their closet and drawers. There are the clothes that fit now, the clothes that fit when they were on their last diet, and perhaps the clothes they hope to fit into again someday.

Take a survey of your wardrobe. Do you have clothes that no longer fit? Consider giving them away or storing them out of sight for now. Do you have enough clothes that fit at your current size? If not, based on your budget, do your best to make sure you have garments that fit the body you have now, as what you wear impacts how you feel during the day.

Fortunately, while it's not perfect, there's a much greater selection of clothes in larger sizes than there's been in the past. Spend some time looking at stores that carry your size, either in person or online. You may want to take advantage of the sales that come at the end of each season or check out a local thrift store. Notice what styles and patterns appeal to you. There's no shame in needing to alter clothes or use button or bra extenders.

Even if you don't want to invest a lot of money in a new wardrobe, it's important to have some outfits that fit you at this time. You may not be sure where your weight will land as you heal your relationship with food, and you deserve to wear clothes that fit you and feel comfortable in the body you have now!

Let Go of the Scale

A familiar feature of diet culture is the need to weigh yourself in the hopes of moving the number down. Dieters often weigh themselves every day, or even multiple times per day. This ritual may involve taking off clothes and jewelry, going to the bathroom, or moving the scale to another spot—anything to see a lower number! Where the number lands can determine if it's going to be a "good" day or a "bad" day.

How do you feel when you get on the scale if the number goes up? Have you ever felt defeated and responded by reaching for food with a sense of "it doesn't matter anyway"? Eating to quell those emotions is perfectly understandable. Food might be the best way you have to help yourself in that moment.

Conversely, how do you feel when the number goes down? Chances are you feel happy, since that's why you're dieting in the first place. But have you ever noticed that after a period of deprivation that resulted in weight loss, you feel like you deserve a reward and respond by going to food? It makes sense, given that deprivation. When you've been undereating to lose weight, your body really does need the nourishment that comes from food.

The takeaway message here? Consider putting away or getting rid of your scale. The scale is an external object that you're giving power to measure your worthiness, and it prevents you from developing a nourishing and pleasurable relationship with food. You deserve to feel worthy in the body you have now.

Make Your Home a Refuge

Take a survey of your home and notice any books, magazines, or other products that promote diet culture. Common items include cookbooks based on diet plans, self-help books on weight loss, magazines with ads for diet plans or that display thin bodies only, and kitchen devices used to weigh and measure food.

Consider removing these items from your home environment and throwing them out. While it's great to donate, when it comes to products supporting dieting and weight loss, we prefer to throw them in the trash or recycling bin so others aren't inundated with these messages. You may also consider replacing these items with books, magazines, and other products that promote body acceptance and diversity.

Remember that the messages you absorb day in and day out impact the way you feel about your body. While you can't control all of the spaces you spend time in, notice how it feels to make your home a place of refuge from diet culture.

Take Stock of Your Social Media

The power of social media is indisputable. Reflect on the types of social media content that you currently view. Do you follow lifestyle influencers who tout the latest wellness hacks for weight loss? What about fitness accounts that promise to give you the body you've always wanted in 30 days or less?

When you see messages on social media that promote weight loss and restrictive eating, or that only display thinner bodies, how do you feel?

_____

_____

_____

_____

When you see messages that promote body acceptance, attuned eating, and a wide range of body sizes, how do you feel?

_____

_____

_____

_____

Let go of social media that's based on diet culture values and replace it with social media that's body positive. As you learn of more resources you can jot them down here.

_____

_____

_____

_____

You may also want to consider taking a social media break. If you try it, use this space to note how it feels.

_____

_____

_____

_____

Strategies to Integrate Body Acceptance into Daily Life

Live in the Present (in a Fatphobic World)

Many chronic dieters avoid doing things they otherwise would like to do—such as going to the beach, asking someone out on a date, or auditioning for a local theater production—because diet culture has taught us to believe that we are not worthy of pursuing or enjoying these things in the bodies we have now. When you put off your goals and activities until you lose weight, you miss out on the pleasure you deserve to have at any size.

What are some things you've missed out on throughout your life because of the way you (or others) felt about your body?

_____

_____

_____

_____

_____

As you reflect on these examples, we want to acknowledge that the anti-fat bias in our culture means that certain goals and activities are less accessible at higher weights, such as riding a roller coaster when the seats are too small or applying for a job when there is discrimination. Use compassion and discernment as you consider what is possible for you to live more fully in the world in the body you have right now.

Make a list of what you've been putting off because of your body size.

_____

_____

_____

_____

From your list, choose a goal or activity that you'd like to work on in the present moment. For example, if you said, "If I were thinner, I would take a dance class," consider how to make that happen. Is there a class offered in your area that focuses on movement, not body size? Or a class that's inclusive of all body sizes? If you prefer to dance in the privacy of your own home, can you find an online dance class? Or put on music at home and dance like nobody's watching (they're not!)? If you're in a higher-weight body, it's important to stay compassionate with yourself as you consider ways to feel safe when you stop putting activities on hold.

Use this space to identify the next steps you can take to put the activity you chose into action.

_____

_____

_____

_____

As you consider the possibility of living more fully in the world in the body you have now, keep in mind that sometimes people's reluctance to pursue their interests is related to core emotional issues. For example, Craig believed that he was putting off dating because of his body size, but when he explored this issue in therapy, he realized that he was frightened of intimate relationships after being abandoned by his father at age five. Craig realized that losing weight wouldn't solve his lack of trust in relationships. This enabled him to focus on the core issue of attachment rather than hooking his fear onto his body and blaming it.

Diet culture teaches us to focus on the pursuit of thinness as a primary means to solve complex emotional issues. Do you think there are any core issues that you've hooked onto your body size?

_____

_____

_____

_____

_____

Take in the Good

Just as you're learning to collect attuned eating experiences that feel good in your body, you can also collect other positive experiences that make you feel good or comfortable in your body. This can include the pleasurable feel of warm water during a shower, the strength of your legs on a hike, or the pleasant sensation of a morning stretch. Or perhaps it's the feeling of sand under your feet at the beach or the soothing coolness of lotion on your skin.

To help you take in the good from these experiences, we've adapted the following visualization, originally created by Rick Hanson (2009), which asks you to think of a time when you felt good *in* your body. Please note that this is a different request than thinking about a time when you felt good *about* your body because of the way it looked from the outside.

Feeling Good in Your Body

To begin, close your eyes, if that's comfortable for you, and think of a time when you felt good in your body. Savor the experience as you hold it in your attention for the next 20 or 30 seconds. Soften and open to the experience, letting it fill your mind and your body. Now, if it feels safe, let it seep even deeper into your body, perhaps as a warm glow spreading through your chest. When you feel ready, open your eyes and notice how you feel.

We encourage you to practice this visualization technique anytime you need a reminder of the goodness you can feel in your body. According to Hanson (2009), any single instance of taking in the good will usually make a difference, but the longer you can hold it in awareness—and the more emotionally stimulating it is—the more you will rewire this new way of thinking into your brain. Over time, those little differences will add up, gradually weaving positive experiences into the fabric of your brain and your whole being.

Body image healing is a journey, not a destination. As you find ways to feel more at home in your body, you're still likely to have moments that feel challenging, such as when you hear an ad for the latest diet product, notice that a friend or colleague has lost weight, or experience emotional distress. Part of this process is finding new ways to respond to negative thoughts that come from diet culture messages, as well as letting go of your own internalized weight stigma. You can support the concept of body positivity and still find that you struggle at times.

Clinician's Corner

As a member of the same diet culture that shapes your clients' attitudes and views about their bodies, you've likely learned the same messages that lead to negative body image. The good news is that you don't have to love your own body to be able to help your clients feel more at home in theirs. At the same time, understanding the inherent diversity of body shapes and sizes, accepting the dismal failure rate of weight loss plans, and encouraging respect and care for all bodies are essential components for helping clients cultivate a more positive body image.

In this chapter, we've offered a variety of activities to help clients feel more at home in their bodies. But that doesn't mean your role is to "fix" your client's body image with a can-do attitude. Sometimes, the most helpful intervention is to hold space with a client to talk about their experience. One way to do that is to say, "Help me understand what it's like to be in your body."

As the client shares their body distress, you can listen on multiple levels. What have they internalized about body size? Where did they learn those messages? Who benefited from the client believing these messages? Are there core issues they've learned to hook onto their body?

For clients who are afraid of becoming fat, what have they been taught about worthiness and weight? For clients who are a higher weight, what are the real challenges they face when they sit in an airplane seat, go to the doctor, or decide to begin dating? The weight stigma out in the world that leads higher-weight clients to be shamed and harmed is real. No amount of body positivity on your client's part will solve those issues, which we'll address in later chapters.

We find that exposing clients to books and articles written about body image and body acceptance, along with podcasts and social media accounts meant to educate and support people of all sizes, are empowering as clients try to unlearn diet culture. If you struggle with your own body image, these resources can benefit you personally as well as professionally.

Use this space to create a list of body image resources that you might want to share with clients. (The resources section at the end of this book is a great place to start!)

_____

_____

_____

_____

_____

As you work with clients to cultivate a healthier body image, the hope is that they will feel more at home in their bodies so they can end their preoccupation with weight, take care of their needs to the extent possible given their life circumstances, and live more fully in the world. We wish that for you too.

Part 3

Finding Solutions

CHAPTER 7

Reconsidering Weight and Health

We exist in a culture that teaches us from an early age that thin is "good" and fat is "bad." We're told that in order to be healthy and live as long as possible, staying thin and pursuing weight loss are of the utmost importance—and "health" is frequently invoked to justify anti-fat bias. These messages are woven into the fabric of our society and perpetuate weight stigma.

In this chapter, we'll explore myths about weight and health, consider the impact of weight stigma on health, and offer strategies to support your health no matter your size. We'll start by asking you to reflect on your own attitudes and language related to body size.

Exploring Your Attitudes Toward Body Size

Take a moment to visualize a thinner body and a fatter body. Without censoring yourself, think about the adjectives you associate with each type of body. What do you notice about your associations?

If you had mostly positive associations with the thinner body and mostly negative associations with the fatter one, then you carry (either explicitly or implicitly) the anti-fat attitudes that are typical in our diet culture.

Use this space to write about any thoughts or feelings that come up for you during this exercise.

_____

_____

_____

_____

_____

This is meant to be an awareness-raising exercise. If you discover that you have an anti-fat bias—and you feel bad about that—we want to assure you that you're not alone. As Emily Nagoski (2015) explains in *Come as You Are*, many people have been exposed to these toxic anti-fat attitudes from their family and their culture: "No one asked your permission before they started planting the toxic crap. They didn't wait until you could give consent and then say, 'Would it be okay with you if we planted the seeds of body self-criticism and sexual shame?' Chances are, they just planted the same things that were planted in their gardens, and it never even occurred to them to plant something different" (p. 155).

Therefore, if you noticed that your associations regarding the thinner versus fatter body were based on stereotypes, judgments, and assumptions, use self-compassion to remind yourself that we've all learned these messages and that they can be challenged. And if you found that your associations didn't match the typical stereotypes, we want to applaud you for the work you've likely done to reach this place of greater neutrality toward body size.

The Language of Body Size

Take a moment to think about the language that diet culture uses to talk about body size. Whenever you go to the doctor for an annual checkup, they likely calculate your body mass index (BMI), with people at higher weights typically described as "overweight" or "obese." These numbers and labels usually increase the shame people feel about their bodies. Before we ask you how you prefer to describe your own body size, consider the following information about BMI, as well as the terms *obese* and *overweight*, and note your reactions.

Body Mass Index

BMI is a mathematical equation based on weight and height. It was developed by Adolphe Quetelet, a Belgian mathematician, statistician, and astronomer, who never intended this calculation to be used as a determinant of individual health. Rather, it was a measure meant to be applied to different populations in search of figuring out the "ideal" body type.

Just as the average family might have 2.3 children (the statistic changes constantly), no one actually has .3 of a child! Likewise, BMI is not an accurate statistic when applied to an individual. In fact, it turns out that if you only use BMI to decide who is healthy and who is unhealthy, you incorrectly label 54 million adults as unhealthy (Tomiyama et al., 2016).

It's also important to note that Quetelet developed BMI using the young white male as the ideal body type. It never took into consideration the bodies of women or people of other races and ethnicities—or, for that matter, the fact that the very concept of an ideal body type is a myth. In her book *Fearing the Black Body*, sociologist Sabrina Strings (2019) describes how anti-fat bias was born out of racist beliefs that saw Black people as "out of control" with food and sex, as part of a justification for enslavement.

"Obesity"

Obesity is a shaming word. In 2013, the American Medical Association declared "obesity" to be a disease, against the advice of their own scientific advisory board. This means that anyone who falls into the obese category is considered to be diseased *regardless* of their actual health status. We've heard stories from people whose bloodwork for markers such as cholesterol and diabetes have come back in the normal range, yet they were told to repeat the test because it was unbelievable to the health care provider that someone at their size could have normal readings. One client reported that his doctor said, "You're the healthiest fat person I know," yet insisted it was still essential to focus on weight loss for health.

"Overweight"

The term *overweight* suggests that there's a correct weight to be, and anyone above this weight is wrong. But who gets to decide what the correct weight is for a particular body? In the 1990s, the National Institutes of Health lowered the cutoffs for the BMI categories, causing millions of people to go to bed at a "normal" weight and wake up the next day "overweight."

The point is that language matters. As you think about what words you might use to describe your body size, consider the following:

- **Higher weight:** We use this term throughout the workbook as a neutral descriptor of body size; it simply indicates that people fall at higher weights and lower weights.

- **Fat:** This term has been used to shame and hurt people, so it may feel uncomfortable or painful to use this adjective to describe yourself if you are at a higher weight. It's important to note that within size accepting communities, the word *fat* has been reclaimed as a neutral term to be used in the same way as other adjectives (e.g., "I'm tall," "I'm short," "I'm thin," "I'm fat"). Reclaiming the word *fat* is similar to the way other marginalized communities have reclaimed words, such as the word *queer* in the LGBTQIA+ community, and it allows fat people to take back their identity in a positive way.

What words do you, or would you prefer to, use to describe your body? How do you feel as you write and think about these descriptors?

_____

_____

_____

_____

_____

_____

A Note About the Phrase "I Feel Fat"

Although this phrase is commonly used in diet culture, fatness is not, in fact, a feeling. When people say, "I feel fat," they often do so instead of identifying and expressing the distressing emotions underlying their experience (e.g., feeling ashamed, anxious, or lonely). Unfortunately, this promotes further weight stigma.

Myths About Weight and Health*

Given the prevalence of news stories and advice that equate thinness with good health, it makes sense that many people believe they must lose weight to be healthy and live a long life. At the same time, there's a wealth of research showing that the relationship between weight and health is not what it seems and that weight is actually a poor indicator of health. Furthermore, the pursuit of weight loss can lead to behaviors that actually worsen health.

Here are three common myths regarding weight:

- Higher weights mean higher mortality rates.

- Higher weights mean more health problems.

- The best way to live longer and healthier is to pursue weight loss through dieting.

In the following section, we'll examine these myths in greater detail and work to dispel the notion that weight loss is a prerequisite for health.

Changing Opinions on "Obesity"

Over the years, several well-respected authors have explained how they changed their minds about the conventional belief that "obesity" is intrinsically harmful. Paul Campos (2004), author of *The Obesity Myth*, explained that when he began his research, he assumed that high weight was such a serious health risk that it was indisputable. Yet after reading hundreds of scientific papers and interviewing numerous experts, he found that "almost everything the government and media were saying about weight and weight control were either grossly distorted or completely untrue" (p. xvi).

Similarly, sociologist J. Eric Oliver (2006), author of *Fat Politics*, changed his mind about body size after realizing that claims about "obesity" were not supported by good evidence: "Based on the statistics, most of the charges saying obesity caused various diseases or that obesity caused thousands of deaths were simply not supported. Yet consistently, these pseudofindings were promulgated as fact" (p. x).

Finally, Gina Kolata (2007), a *New York Times* science reporter and the author of *Rethinking Thin*, noted, "Why is it that the scientific truths about obesity are so often unknown or ignored by anti-obesity crusaders and by struggling dieters? Why is it that even obesity fighters . . . either do not know what science has learned or choose to ignore or deny it?" (p. 188).

---

* As we explore this topic, please note we use the terms *obesity* and *overweight* when they are used in the research. We use quotation marks as a reminder that these are not descriptors we endorse.

Weight and Longevity

Despite the long-held misconception that higher weight is associated with higher mortality rates, research published in the *Journal of the American Medical Association* says otherwise. In particular, a systematic review by Katherine Flegal and colleagues (2013), which analyzed the results of numerous other studies, confirmed the following: People who fall into the "overweight" BMI category have the lowest mortality risk, while people in the "normal" weight category and lower end of the "obese" category have the same risk (which is just slightly higher than those in the "overweight" category). People at the higher end of the "obese" category have a slightly higher mortality rate, while people in the "underweight" category have the highest mortality rate. If you imagine a U-shaped curve, it's the people at the outer edges that have the highest mortality rates.

Just as it was difficult for people to shift their belief from "the earth is flat" to "the earth is round" in the time of Galileo, most people find it challenging to believe that being at a higher weight doesn't automatically mean a shorter life.

When you think about the possibility that the fears around weight and longevity have been overblown, how do you feel?

_____

_____

_____

_____

_____

_____

Weight, Health, and Physical Fitness

Although it is commonly believed that people who are of "normal" weight must be healthy (and that people who are "overweight" must be unhealthy), physical fitness level is a much better predictor of health outcomes than weight alone. For example, a recent study by professors of exercise physiology at Arizona State University found that people who focus on the pursuit of weight loss often get caught in the futile cycle of weight-loss-and-regain, and they do not achieve any health benefits (Gaesser & Angadi, 2021). Conversely, when people take a weight-neutral approach, where weight loss is not an indicator of their success, physical activity and fitness offer health benefits *regardless* of whether their weight goes up, goes down, or stays the same.

We do want to recognize that this research is based on able-bodied people and that there may be other circumstances, such as living in a neighborhood that is unsafe for walking, that make it difficult or impossible to add physical activity into your life. You may also be healing from a disordered relationship with exercise, in which case the best approach for you might be to take a break from physical activity for now. If physical activity has been part of the diet cycle for you, it may take some time to reclaim movement as self-care.

Additionally, there is no moral obligation to pursue health in this way. What we want to point out, however, is that so much energy goes into insisting that people pursue weight loss, which has no research to demonstrate long-term success for the majority of people, while movement can make a significant difference in supporting health.

When you think about the possibility that a behavior such as physical activity can have a more positive effect on health than weight loss, how do you feel?

_____

_____

_____

_____

_____

_____

As you reconsider your own beliefs about weight and health, remember that correlation doesn't equal causation. For example, consider the known fact that a man who is bald is at higher risk of cardiovascular disease. Let's imagine giving him a toupee so he's no longer bald, with the idea that this action will lower his risk for heart problems. Sound ridiculous? That's because there's a third factor at play here. Some men have higher testosterone levels that are responsible for both a greater chance of baldness *and* greater risk of cardiovascular disease. It's a correlation, not a causation. Likewise, consider that weight may be correlated with health when there are other factors at play.

Weight Loss, Yo-Yo Dieting, and Health

In our culture, weight loss recommendations abound, with the message that it's in your best interest to at least try dieting to become thinner. However, as we have discussed, dieting does not result in sustained weight loss for the vast majority of people, not to mention that it may have harmful health consequences. In fact, people who diet are at greater risk of developing eating disorders, which have one of the highest rates of death for mental health conditions.

In her book *Sick Enough*, Jennifer Gaudiani (2019) details the severe, but often undiagnosed, medical conditions that can result from eating disorders, including bone loss, heart and liver damage, and kidney failure. We also know that teens who diet are much more likely to develop BED and to experience depression, low self-esteem, and suicidality *regardless* of their starting weight.

While not everyone who diets develops an eating disorder, most people who pursue weight loss will end up weight cycling because of the high rates of diet failure. Many studies have found that weight cycling—also known as yo-yo dieting—can have negative effects on health. For example, a Harvard alumni study followed men over decades and found that those who stayed at a higher, steady weight lived longer than those whose weight fluctuated up and down (Gaesser, 2002). Similarly, researchers from Columbia University, in conjunction with the American Heart Association, found that more episodes of yo-yo dieting were associated with worse cardiovascular health among women (Byun et al., 2019).

Remember that weight cycling also virtually guarantees higher weights over time. (Again, it's not that there's anything wrong with having a higher-weight body, but as we discussed in chapter 2, the diet cycle changes your physiology.) When that happens, you're blamed for your body size, told you'll suffer ill health as a result, and encouraged to lose weight once again. What a bind!

When you think about the possibility that yo-yo dieting is associated with worse health outcomes than being at a steady, higher weight, how do you feel?

_____

_____

_____

_____

_____

A Weight-Inclusive Framework

Although weight-management approaches claim to improve health outcomes via weight loss, there's (ironically) no way to even prove this claim is true because most people who lose weight are unable to keep it off long enough to become part of a study.

The alternative to the weight-management approach is to learn about what's known as a weight-neutral or weight-inclusive framework, such as the Health at Every Size® (HAES®) paradigm. These frameworks look at factors beyond weight that impact health, don't use the number on the scale to assess health, and recognize the impact of fat shaming, weight stigma, and other social determinants on health. A weight-inclusive framework promotes behaviors that support your physical and emotional well-being, like exercise, sleep, nutrition, stress management, and social connection. It also means that health providers offer higher-weight patients the same strategies and treatments that they offer to their thinner patients.

To begin shifting toward a weight-inclusive approach, take a survey of behaviors that you currently practice in the name of health, whether it's the types of foods you eat, the supplements you take, or the types of exercise you engage in. Note whether you would still practice each specific behavior if you weren't pursuing weight loss, and whether it's truly sustainable, by circling yes or no.

Behavior	For the Purpose of Weight Loss?	Sustainable?
	Yes or No	Yes or No
	Yes or No	Yes or No
	Yes or No	Yes or No
	Yes or No	Yes or No
	Yes or No	Yes or No
	Yes or No	Yes or No
	Yes or No	Yes or No

If you listed any behaviors that are for the purpose of weight loss or that are not sustainable, consider letting them go. Although you may believe that you're giving up and doomed to be in poor health if you don't pursue weight loss, rest assured that there are all kinds of ways to take care of your body at any size.

The following is a list of positive, sustainable self-care practices that will support your body without a focus on weight loss. This is not an exhaustive list, nor are these meant to be new rules or guidelines. Instead, notice how you feel toward each category, whether these practices are accessible to you, and whether they are reminiscent of the diet mindset for you.

Exercise

Unfortunately, exercise has become intricately entwined with the diet mindset. You're "good" when you do it and "bad" when you don't. You may use exercise as punishment for having the "wrong" body, even exercising to the point where it feels physically or emotionally painful. You may feel guilty when you don't exercise "enough." You may make a resolution to exercise at the start of each New Year, only to find yourself stopping completely when you miss a day or two of your promised exercise plan.

If you have negative associations with the word *exercise*, consider using the terms *movement* or *activity* to describe how your body wants to move.

Think about a time when you enjoyed movement. Go back to childhood if necessary as you remember some experiences of moving your body that felt enjoyable.

_____

_____

_____

_____

To help you unhook physical activity from the pursuit of weight loss, make a list of reasons that someone might choose to be physically active in ways that aren't related to body size. For example, moving their body might be a way to help them achieve flexibility, mobility, strength, health benefits, social connection, pleasure, or more. List possible reasons here:

_____

_____

_____

_____

Finally, remind yourself that movement is not an obligation by listing the reasons *you* would like to move your body, including the types of movement that would feel best to you.

I would like to engage in some movement because: _____

_____

The type of movement that would feel best to my body is: _____

_____

In order to get started I need to: _____

_____

If you find that you'd like to add movement to your routine, but you can't seem to get going, or your relationship with movement feels compulsive, approach your situation with compassion and curiosity:

- How is the part of you that's stuck in the diet mindset trying to help or protect you?

- If you're overexercising, what would happen if you slowed down or took a break?

- If you're at a higher weight, stigma can be a factor in putting yourself out there. Can you check out resources in person or online for instructors whose offerings are for those in larger bodies?

- If you experience chronic pain or a disability, are there ways to move your body that feel supportive to you?

_____

_____

_____

_____

_____

Sleep

Getting a good night's sleep is vital for your mental and physical health, but many people are sleep deprived. Sleep experts recommend that adults get at least seven hours of sleep per night, with some people needing as many as ten hours each night. If you're not getting enough sleep, reflect on whether it is possible to take any steps at this time in your life to improve your sleep quality, such as having a consistent bedtime routine, keeping your bedroom dark, reducing exposure to screens in the evening, and limiting caffeine intake later in the day.

There are other factors that can interfere with sleep, such as anxiety or sleep apnea. If these situations apply to you, consider working with a health professional to seek strategies and treatments that will leave you feeling more rested.

If there are reasons for sleep deprivation that are beyond your control, such as working a night shift, working multiple jobs, or having young children who wake up during the night, consider offering yourself compassion for the impact that has on you. Use this space to reflect on your sleep habits and any next steps that you want to take at this time.

_____

_____

_____

_____

_____

_____

Gentle Nutrition

As you make peace with food, gentle nutrition allows you to think about how different foods support your body. In general, think about what you want to add to your diet, rather than what diet culture tells you to eliminate. In chapter 8, we'll explore this concept in more depth.

Stress Management

Although stress is a natural part of life, when you're in a state of stress day in and day out, it takes a toll on your body and mind. In chapter 4, we introduced a simple diaphragmatic breathing exercise and a visualization technique to help you move out of a state of sympathetic nervous activation and into a state of relaxation. The following are some additional calming practices you might want to try to manage the effects of stress:

- Engage in progressive muscle relaxation

- Practice yoga

- Try aromatherapy

- Get or give yourself a massage

- Buy yourself some flowers

- Spend time in nature

- Engage in hobbies

- Enjoy coloring books or jigsaw puzzles

- Add any other activities you find relaxing: _____

_____

_____

While these types of practices will not solve all the stress you may experience, including the effects of trauma and marginalization, they can help your body mitigate its impact. Consider also searching for mindfulness apps, books, or local offerings and make a list of ideas to further explore.

_____

_____

_____

_____

Social Connection

As human beings, we are wired to connect with each other. Our need for social connection is perhaps as fundamental as our need for food, shelter, clothing, and other essentials. In fact, studies consistently show that social isolation leads to poorer physical and mental health, while positive social relationships and frequent social contacts are protective for our physical and emotional well-being (Mineo, 2017; NIH, 2017).

Here are some ideas to help you seek out or maintain social connections:

- Spend time with people you love

- Pursue creative outlets

- Join a book group

- Take a class

- Volunteer

- Play team sports

- Take part in a religious or other community

- Add any other activities you find helpful for social connection: _____

_____

_____

What experiences give you the greatest sense of belonging?

_____

_____

_____

_____

If you would like to feel a greater sense of belonging, what is your next step to find or create this experience?

_____

_____

_____

_____

Now that you've learned ways to support your physical and emotional well-being that don't involve weight loss, are there any other positive, sustainable behaviors that will support your body? Think about how you can add these behaviors in a way that works with your current life.

_____

_____

_____

_____

_____

_____

Weight, Stigma, and Health

The Social Determinants of Health

When people talk about the relationship between weight and health, it's often looked at from a stance of personal responsibility. *You* are deemed responsible for how much you weigh and how this affects your health. Your weight, in turn, may be blamed for a variety of health conditions. Common advice is to cut back on certain types of foods and increase exercise in order to lose weight and be healthy.

Although health behaviors seem to account for 25 to 30 percent of population health outcomes (Park et al., 2015), they're not the only influence, as there are numerous factors on a population level that can affect health. Some of these social determinants include:

- Lack of access to adequate medical care or medications due to cost, availability, weight bias, or other forms of discrimination

- Chronic stress due to job or food insecurity

- Environmental factors that increase exposure to pollutants, such as poor air quality

When it comes to health and weight, it turns out that your zip code is a better predictor of outcomes than your weight. For example, people living in neighborhoods with high crime rates are less likely to feel safe walking outdoors. People living in areas with few grocery stores have less access to fresh fruits and vegetables, which are also much more expensive to purchase. People who have lower incomes usually have less access to medical care. Additional factors can exacerbate these social disparities, including a person's race, ethnicity, gender identity, sexual orientation, ability, age, and body size, as individuals from marginalized groups face greater forms of oppression and discrimination.

Weight Stigma

Weight stigma occurs anytime you feel you're treated unfairly because of your body size. You may experience weight stigma in the workplace or job market, at the doctor's office, or in your interactions with any number of individuals and institutions. Many of our clients, especially those at higher weights, dread appointments with medical providers because of the shaming they experience now or have in the past. Their providers blame their weight for all their health concerns, prescribe weight loss (even despite the existence of an eating disorder), or don't take symptoms seriously.

Whether or not health professionals have made explicit comments about your weight, you may have experienced less overt expressions of weight stigma. The act of being weighed can trigger body shame. Weight stigma can affect your health when you don't get an accurate diagnosis, or you put off doctor's appointments to avoid being shamed. It's understandable to want to protect yourself from weight stigma in medical settings. At the same time, seeing your doctor on a regular basis is an important part of caring for yourself, and you deserve to receive respectful care.

If you have experienced shaming and stigma with medical providers, here are some ideas about how to advocate for yourself at a doctor's visit:

- If your doctor prescribes weight loss for your health condition, ask them if they ever see this health condition in their thinner patients. (Hint: The answer will be yes.) Let them know you'd like the same treatments and strategies they offer their thinner patients with similar symptoms, such as a referral to physical therapy if you're in pain or medication for high cholesterol.

- Check out the *HAES® Health Sheets*, which offer blame-free, shame-free explanations of common medical conditions, co-authored by an internal medicine physician: haeshealthsheets. com.

- Check out these *Don't Weigh Me* cards, which you can give to your doctor: more-love.org /resources/free-dont-weigh-me-cards.

You can also use the following space to write a letter to your doctor or other health provider about what you'd like them to understand when it comes to your history and experiences with dieting, weight, shame, health, or self-care. Some of our clients have found it helpful to send this letter in advance or to hand it to their doctor at the time of their appointment—it's up to you!

_____

_____

_____

_____

_____

_____

_____

_____

_____

It's important to acknowledge that fat shaming at the doctor's office can make it hard to speak up for yourself. Even if you can advocate for yourself, it doesn't guarantee that you'll get the care you need and deserve. While you may think this is evidence as to why you should pursue weight loss, remember that there are no proven ways to lose weight and keep it off.

Instead, we think it's important to locate the problem where it belongs: It's not your body that's the problem, it's the anti-fat bias that exists in our culture. Remember, no matter how far you've come in cultivating a more positive body image, these strategies don't make you immune from the weight stigma that's so prevalent in our culture. The way you are treated because of your body size isn't your fault, but it still impacts you. Ultimately, changing the way people think about weight, and changing the institutions that uphold weight bias, will lead to creating a world that treats all bodies with respect.

We encourage you to explore strategies and find community (more about that in chapter 9) to manage and reject weight stigma to the extent possible for you.

Misconceptions About a Weight-Inclusive Approach

As you consider a weight-inclusive approach or discuss it with important people in your life, you may find that they have some misconceptions about this approach. Remember, making a major shift in thinking is tough! Here are some common myths about a weight-inclusive framework, as developed by Judith and her colleague Carmen Cool, and counterpoints to these myths.

- **Myth 1: A weight-inclusive approach means that all higher-weight people can be healthy.**
  A weight-inclusive approach means that people of all sizes deserve to pursue, and have equal access to, strategies and treatments that support their bodies in achieving optimal health as they define it. Health is a continuum: There are people at higher weights who are healthy and those

who are not healthy, just as there are people at lower weights who are healthy and those who are not healthy. A weight-inclusive approach also acknowledges the role that stigma, bias, and oppression play in a person's health.

- **Myth 2: A weight-inclusive approach is against weight loss.** A weight-inclusive approach is against the pursuit of weight loss given the dismal failure rate of diets and the physical and emotional harm that results. It encourages people to take care of their bodies, and if weight changes occur, it is a side effect rather than the goal. It does not use weight loss as a measure of success.

- **Myth 3: A weight-inclusive approach is only relevant to people at higher weights.** A weight-inclusive approach is an important framework for people of all sizes. At its core, this approach seeks to end stigma toward people based on body size. It acknowledges that people across the weight spectrum feel the effects of weight stigma, fear of fat, and diet culture. This approach can help people take the focus off weight and, instead, focus on living their best life as they define it.

When you can counter these myths with education and understanding, you might find that people become more open and accepting of this approach. Although we have no doubt that you'll continue to be bombarded by messages that tell you thinness is a prerequisite for health, we hope this chapter gives you alternative ways to think about your own weight and health from a place of strength and healing. And if you find that, at times, you still wonder, "But what if I *really* need to lose weight for my health?" we gently ask you to consider this quote from Christy's book *Anti-Diet* (Harrison, 2019):

> Until all research can control for weight cycling and weight stigma, we can't say that being at the higher end of the BMI spectrum *causes* any health conditions—even if higher weights are *associated* with these health conditions. Remember that statistical golden rule: Correlation does not equal causation. Moreover, even if weight *did* have some causal effect on people's health (which is possible—but again, we can't know until we control for weight stigma and weight cycling), we don't have a known way for more than a tiny fraction of people to lose weight and keep it off permanently. (pp. 145–146)

Clinician's Corner

If you picked up this workbook because you already use a weight-inclusive approach with your clients, that's terrific! We hope our resource supports your ongoing work. But if a weight-inclusive approach is new to you, the information in this chapter can be a lot to take in—for you as well as your clients. Take your time as you consider the research related to weight and health and use it to inform your clinical work. As you see articles in the media or come across studies that promote the pursuit of weight loss, be sure to ask yourself the following:

- Does the study show that participants' weight loss is sustainable over a five-year period? Keep in mind that weight regain often begins at the one-year mark and speeds up over the following years. Many studies have data that is less than one year old, so it cannot be considered accurate.

- Do the researchers have any conflicts of interest? For example, "obesity" researchers often have ties to pharmaceutical companies that are creating drugs to produce weight loss.

- What are the side effects of the intervention?

It can be challenging to stay on top of the latest research so that you can feel comfortable in your recommendations to your clients. Find online groups or subscribe to podcasts or newsletters that will help you keep learning about issues related to weight, health, and stigma.

We also encourage you to complete the following prompts, which can help you consider your current attitudes toward health and weight and what you are likely bringing to the clinical setting. Set your alarm and spend three to five minutes writing your response to each prompt without censoring yourself. Don't worry about spelling or grammar—just let the words flow! Afterward, reflect on your responses and see where you're at when it comes to thinking about weight and health.

When I think about implementing a weight-inclusive framework, I:

_____

_____

_____

_____

The most exciting part of a weight-inclusive framework is:

_____

_____

_____

_____

The biggest obstacle I see in using a weight-inclusive framework is:

_____

_____

_____

_____

In order to use a weight-inclusive framework in my own life, I need to:

_____

_____

_____

_____

Another tool that may be of interest to you is the *Assessing Your Size Attitudes* assessment, which appears in the book *Beyond a Shadow of a Diet* (Matz & Frankel, 2004). This tool can be used to evaluate your support for the health and well-being of people at higher weights.

Assessing Your Size Attitudes*

Use the following scale to indicate the frequency of each behavior.

1 = Never   2 = Rarely   3 = Occasionally   4 = Frequently   5 = Daily

How often do you:

1. Make negative comments about your fatness	1 2 3 4 5
2. Make negative comments about someone else's fatness	1 2 3 4 5
3. Directly or indirectly support the assumption that no one should be fat	1 2 3 4 5
4. Disapprove of fatness (in general)	1 2 3 4 5
5. Say or assume that someone is "looking good" because they have lost weight	1 2 3 4 5
6. Say something that presumes a fat person wants to lose weight	1 2 3 4 5
7. Say something that presumes a fat person should lose weight	1 2 3 4 5
8. Say something that presumes fat people eat too much	1 2 3 4 5

* Excerpt from *Making Peace with Food* by Susan Kano. Copyright © 1989 by Susan Kano. Reprinted by permission of HarperCollins Publishers Inc., New York, NY.

9. Admire or approve of someone for losing weight	1 2 3 4 5
10. Disapprove of someone for gaining weight	1 2 3 4 5
11. Assume that something is wrong when someone gains weight	1 2 3 4 5
12. Admire weight loss	1 2 3 4 5
13. Admire rigidly controlled eating	1 2 3 4 5
14. Admire compulsive or excessive exercising	1 2 3 4 5
15. Tease or admonish someone about their eating habits or choices	1 2 3 4 5
16. Criticize someone's eating to a third person ("So-and-so eats way too much junk")	1 2 3 4 5
17. Discuss food in terms of "good" and "bad"	1 2 3 4 5
18. Talk about "being good" and "being bad" in reference to eating behavior	1 2 3 4 5
19. Talk about calories (in the usual dieter's fashion)	1 2 3 4 5
20. Say something that presumes being thin is better (or more attractive) than being fat	1 2 3 4 5
21. Comment that you don't wear a certain style because "it makes you look fat"	1 2 3 4 5
22. Comment that you love certain clothing because "it makes you look thin"	1 2 3 4 5
23. Say something that presumes fatness is unattractive	1 2 3 4 5
24. Participate in a "fat joke" by telling one or laughing or smiling at one	1 2 3 4 5
25. Support the diet industry by buying their services or products	1 2 3 4 5
26. Undereat or exercise obsessively to maintain an unnaturally low weight	1 2 3 4 5
27. Say something that presumes being fat is unhealthy	1 2 3 4 5
28. Say something that presumes being thin is healthy	1 2 3 4 5
29. Encourage someone to let go of guilt	1 2 3 4 5

30. Encourage or admire self-acceptance, self-appreciation, and self-love	1 2 3 4 5
31. Encourage someone to feel good about their body as is	1 2 3 4 5
32. Openly admire a fat person's appearance	1 2 3 4 5
33. Openly admire a fat person's character, personality, or actions	1 2 3 4 5
34. Oppose or challenge fattism verbally	1 2 3 4 5
35. Oppose or challenge fattism in writing	1 2 3 4 5
36. Challenge or voice disapproval of a "fat joke"	1 2 3 4 5
37. Challenge myths about fatness and eating	1 2 3 4 5
38. Compliment ideas, behavior, and character more often than appearance	1 2 3 4 5
39. Support organizations that advance fat acceptance (with your time or money)	1 2 3 4 5

Behaviors 1–28 are unhelpful or harmful to a weight-inclusive approach, so look over areas that need improvement and strive to avoid these and similar behaviors in the future. Behaviors 29–39 support size acceptance, so reread any items you marked "never" or "rarely," and make a list of realistic goals for increasing your supportive behavior.

Over the years, workshop participants who completed this assessment have made statements such as "I don't judge other people, but I'm still really hard on myself," "I didn't realize I thought these things," and "I thought I was further along in letting go of my biases, but I realize I still have more to unlearn." We encourage you to hold compassion toward yourself as you reflect on your responses and, at the same time, to make a commitment to work on your own internalized weight stigma.

If you work in an organization, consider policies that support weight diversity instead of those that uphold weight stigma. If you have colleagues who are steeped in diet culture, consider sharing some of what you're learning with them. Perhaps you can even offer a staff training on some of the topics discussed in this workbook.

In addition to working with clients to advocate for themselves and to use the strategies offered in this chapter, you may offer to be an advocate for them by speaking with their health care professional. Explain their diet history and how recommendations for restriction may lead to disordered eating. This can be of great support to clients in getting treatment that supports their total well-being. The *HAES Health Sheets* mentioned earlier in this chapter are an excellent resource too.

CHAPTER 8

Health, Wellness, and Nutrition

As we've discussed throughout this workbook, recovery from binge eating, emotional eating, and chronic dieting involves learning to let go of diet culture rules and tune into internal cues for hunger, fullness, and satisfaction. Healing from these issues means moving away from restrictive diets and moralizing ideas about "good" and "bad" foods. It means challenging diet culture's beliefs about health and wellness, and instead approaching nutrition in a gentle and self-caring way. A peaceful relationship with food is about self-care, not self-control.

But what if you have a health condition that seems to require you to eat certain foods and avoid others—or you're trying to prevent getting one? In this chapter, we'll address these concerns while also helping you stay connected to all the skills and practices you've been learning so far. Indeed, this chapter was designed to build on the rest of the workbook, not to be read in isolation or out of order.

We waited until this point in the workbook to discuss nutrition because we know that most people healing from binge eating, emotional eating, and chronic dieting already have more than enough nutrition information swirling around in their heads. Before adding any more, we needed to try to reduce the noise.

Even if you're itching to get to the point where you can intuitively choose foods that feel good for your body, you probably won't be able to incorporate nutrition information in an attuned way until you've done your best to reject the diet mindset. In fact, if you pursue nutrition too early, you'll likely default to what Christy calls the "Wellness Diet"—the modern manifestation of diet culture that pretends to be all about nutrition and health. The Wellness Diet turns attuned eating into just another diet, with food rules and morality attached to food choices. It's only at the very end of the attuned eating process that you can come back to nutrition in a way that's gentle and self-caring instead of restrictive and self-controlling.

Once you are ready to revisit nutrition from a place of self-care and break down some of the nutrition myths that you picked up in your dieting days, then this chapter is for you. But if at any point you start to relate to this information in a way that feels diet-y—if you become worried about eating the "wrong" things or "too much" of certain foods—we invite you to work on challenging these thoughts by reviewing previous chapters and then revisiting this one.

Reframing Nutrition

Knowing some basic nutrition information can help you manage your energy levels and feel your best, but please remember that nutrition is not the be-all-and-end-all of health—the way it's often portrayed in diet culture. It won't make you live forever or give you a rich and shiny life. It may not even prevent disease, because while eating in a balanced way may (or may not) help lower your risk of some diseases, it doesn't reduce the risk to zero.

You may be surprised to learn that when it comes to modifiable determinants of health, diet and exercise *combined* only account for about 10 percent of health outcomes, while other behaviors such as smoking, alcohol and drug use, and safe sex account for about 20 percent (Hood et al. 2016; Park et al., 2015). Although this research applies to the general population, even at an individual level, nutrition really isn't as central to our health as we've been led to believe. Granted, nutrition is important in the sense that we need to have *enough* food and a wide enough *variety* of foods to keep our bodies satisfied and nourished. But a balanced relationship with food—and a balanced life—is about so much more than just nutrition. It's about connection, relationships, satisfaction, pleasure, and purpose.

Moreover, as we've discussed, social determinants of health are much bigger predictors of disease or well-being than nutrition alone. Job insecurity, discrimination, violence, and lack of access to clean air and medical care can't be fixed by providing people with nutrition education or giving them access to particular types of food. These are larger issues that need to be addressed at the societal and policy levels. Health is about so much more than individual choices.

Another problem with a hyperfocus on nutrition is the risk of developing orthorexia, which, as we discussed previously, is a form of disordered eating that involves an obsession with the health and purity of food. Being too obsessed with eating well and maintaining the identity of a "healthy" person can actually lead to worse overall well-being than being flexible with your eating. In fact, although there are endless debates about the "right" way to eat (and endless studies that ultimately show disappointing results for various diets), the most enduring principles of nutrition are variety and balance.

These principles mean you can enjoy a wide variety of foods, such as pizza, burgers, fries, donuts, and candy, as well as vegetables, fruits, whole grains, and even trendy "wellness" foods like green juices or smoothie bowls, if you genuinely enjoy them. The key to being able to approach nutrition in this balanced and self-compassionate way is to integrate awareness of your internal cues with awareness of gentle nutrition concepts, which we'll work on developing here.

How have you thought about nutrition in the past, and how might you reframe it now? Are there any food rules that you're starting to reconsider?

_____

_____

_____

_____

Eating for Energy

As you may have learned by tuning into your body throughout this workbook, hunger tends to set in a few hours after each time you eat. That's because your body's blood sugar levels reach a low point around that time. Whenever your blood sugar dips into the low side of the "normal" range, your body sends out hunger signals that tell you to eat. And when everything is functioning in the usual way (e.g., you don't have diabetes and you're not overriding your hunger signals through dieting or disordered eating behaviors), the system works beautifully to keep your blood sugar levels stable.

The body is amazing that way. It's keenly sensitive to levels of essential chemicals in our bloodstream, and it works to bring them back into balance. That's called homeostasis, and it works for glucose (blood sugar) as well as for many other chemicals and compounds, like sodium, water, and so on. Blood sugar gives us energy and fuels our bodies to do literally everything, from writing emails to hiking mountains, from cooking meals to launching businesses.

When you're not eating enough overall and your blood sugar reaches very low points (perhaps punctuated by binges or episodes of rebound eating), it's hard to have the sustained energy you need to get things done. You also might feel moody, upset, or erratic, which isn't helpful for your mental well-being. Eating enough throughout the day is a great way to practice self-care because it helps keep your blood sugar levels a bit more stable, thereby helping you feel your best. It may also help reduce the risk of type 2 diabetes (which is a condition in which your body stops being able to regulate blood sugar on its own) and may help you manage diabetes if you already have it.

Eating at subtle signs of hunger, rather than waiting until you're ravenous and "hangry," can help your blood sugar stay relatively stable. (You can review the signs of hunger in chapter 3.) Another way to help keep your blood sugar ebbing and flowing smoothly is to include three key nutrients in your meals and snacks: carbohydrate, protein, and fat. These three components, also known as *macronutrients*, are the building blocks of sustained energy:

- **Carbohydrate** is the quick-acting form of energy that brings your blood sugar up when it's low. If you don't have adequate carbohydrates in a meal or snack, you likely won't feel very energized by the food.

- **Protein** is a medium-length energy source. It takes longer to break down than carbohydrates but less time than fat, and its presence in a meal or snack helps keep your blood sugar stable longer.

- **Fat** is the long-acting form of energy. It further reduces the speed at which your blood sugar rises and takes the longest to break down of the three nutrients mentioned here, contributing to blood sugar stability.

When you hear this information, how does it square with what you've experienced in your own observations of hunger, fullness, and satisfaction?

_____

_____

_____

_____

If hearing the terms *carbohydrate* and *fat* sends you right back to the diet mindset, you might revisit chapter 3 and do the journal activities there. Then you can circle back to this chapter when you're feeling able to keep diet thoughts in their place.

There are endless ways to build a meal or snack with these three components. Carbohydrates include all kinds of grains and grain products (such as rice, pasta, tortillas, and bread) and starchy vegetables (such as potatoes and corn) and help give a meal the power to really satisfy. Protein includes meat, poultry, fish, eggs, cheese, and plant-based options such as tofu or tempeh. Fat includes oil, butter, coconut milk, and a vast array of sauces made with these ingredients.

Cuisines around the world typically include these building blocks in their meals. Can you think of some examples from your own culinary traditions?

_____

_____

_____

_____

Another building block that shows up in cuisines throughout the world is produce—fruits and vegetables. These can be cooked into stews and sauces; served on the side of the main meal of carbs, protein, and fat; or combined with other components in a variety of ways. They add flavor and texture to a dish, such as a satisfying crunch, refreshing notes of acidity, a fiery heat, or other properties that help balance out the meal. Fruits and vegetables provide vitamins and minerals—technically called *micronutrients* because they're physically much smaller than macronutrients and because our need for them is comparatively smaller too.

Contrary to what diet and wellness culture sometimes claim, produce isn't the part of the meal that really satisfies or leads to long-term fullness. Eating very large amounts of fruits and vegetables may temporarily make your stomach feel full, but it can also lead to bloating and discomfort, as well as a lack of satisfaction and hunger relatively soon after a meal. Unfortunately, many people eat produce in ways they don't actually enjoy because of pressure from diet and wellness culture. It would be a lot easier for people to find pleasure in fruits and vegetables if we weren't subjected to these shaming messages.

What are some ways that fruits and vegetables are used in your culinary traditions? What fats, sauces, and cooking methods are used to make them taste delicious?

_____

_____

_____

_____

If you've been treating produce as a "should," what's one thing you can do to make it more pleasurable?

_____

_____

How a Balanced Meal or Snack Feels

You won't be able to create balanced meals and snacks every time you eat, and that's totally okay! But you might notice that they do give you different energy levels than less-balanced options.

To help you reflect on the energizing potential of different meals and snacks, experiment with some of the following variations (or any other options you enjoy) and see if you notice any differences in how long you feel satisfied by each variation, how long it takes to get hungry again, and any other changes in your energy levels and enjoyment of the food. As always, if you find this suggestion triggering, please skip it. It's not worth jeopardizing all your hard work in healing your relationship with food for one workbook activity!

- Toast with jam
- Toast with peanut butter and jam
- Caesar salad with croutons
- Caesar salad with croutons and chicken or tofu
- Caesar salad with croutons, chicken or tofu, and a half sandwich
- Handful of raisins
- Handful of trail mix (fruit and nuts)
- Crackers and fruit
- Crackers and cheese

After trying out any of these food combinations, use this space to record your observations and note any differences in how you feel.

_____

_____

_____

_____

_____

If you notice any differences, remember not to turn your food choices into rules (e.g., "If I'm going to eat crackers, it must *always* be with cheese"). Instead, just use this information to help you in taking care of your needs each day. There will be some times when you'll want to be sustained for several hours, and other times when you'll just want a little something to tide you over for an hour until dinner. Use your reflections from this activity to help you find food options that will fit the bill for each type of situation.

Be sure to keep honoring your desires and tastes in this process and remind yourself that satisfaction is key. Forgive yourself if you're not able to select the "right" option for every situation, because nobody can. Instead, use this activity to gather data and then do the best you can to care for yourself, knowing that there's no possible way to do it "perfectly."

It's Not About "Perfection"

Diet and wellness culture create the illusion that there's a "perfect" and "right" way of eating, and that if we all just ate that way, then the rest of our lives would magically fall into place. But that's just not the case. Barring serious anaphylactic allergies (e.g., a peanut or shellfish allergy), your individual food choices are not matters of life and death. (And even then, there are medical treatments to keep you alive if you do accidentally eat something you're seriously allergic to.)

Wellness culture makes it seem like the key to a long and happy life is knowing each and every chemical and additive in your food, but for most people, that kind of knowledge only leads to fear, overwhelm, and disordered eating. Granted, as we've been discussing, there's value in knowing about basic nutrients to help you build meals and snacks that satisfy you. But even being able to implement this gentle form of nutrition knowledge without having diet culture creep in is a pretty advanced move. And wellness culture's prohibitions on gluten, grains, dairy, certain oils, sugar, and "processed" foods are more likely to make you run yourself ragged with worry than they are to truly help your well-being.

We want to emphasize that the vast majority of people don't have any sort of food allergy or intolerance and don't need to cut out foods or food groups. If you have a genuine food allergy or a diagnosed digestive issue like celiac disease, it's certainly good self-care to honor that. But if not, eliminating foods in the name of digestive health can actually exacerbate disordered eating. Consider honoring the fact that you can be open to all different kinds of foods and that any digestive discomfort or other symptoms you're experiencing are more likely to be a product of dieting and disordered eating behaviors than they are to be an issue with the food itself.

In fact, it turns out that anxiety about particular foods can actually *make* those foods cause digestive discomfort. It's called the nocebo effect, which is the opposite of the placebo effect—the placebo effect is when you believe something is going to make you feel better, so it does, while the nocebo effect is when you believe something is going to make you feel worse, so it does.

The nocebo effect is very powerful, and it's a recognized factor in research on digestive disorders. For example, a landmark 2013 study found that people who identified as having a non-celiac gluten sensitivity actually weren't sensitive to gluten, but they still exhibited a strong nocebo response because of the mere expectation that the researchers were serving them gluten (Biesiekierski et al., 2013).

In addition, digestive disorders can actually be caused by disordered eating, rather than by the foods we eat. For example, up to 98 percent of people with eating disorders have some sort of functional gut disorder (Boyd et al., 2005), which makes complete sense because disordered eating behaviors wreak havoc on the digestive system. If you have a digestive disorder that you suspect might be exacerbated by particular foods, we invite you to consider the role that the diet mindset might be playing in your belief that certain foods cause discomfort and in your desire to eliminate them. Because diet culture demonizes certain foods, it's likely that the nocebo effect will come into play with those foods.

You might also consider the possibility that some lingering disordered eating behaviors could be causing digestive issues. As you work on letting go of those behaviors and making peace with food—*all* foods—you may find that you're able to tolerate certain foods you once thought of as problematic for your digestion. Or you may find that certain foods continue to cause symptoms even as you make peace with food. Even if you have a medically diagnosed digestive disorder, such as Crohn's disease, lactose intolerance, or celiac disease, it's worth teasing apart which of your beliefs about particular foods are coming from a place of self-care and which are coming from the diet mindset.

What About "Medically Necessary" Diets?

Some health conditions might require modifying the way you eat. For example, people with diabetes have trouble regulating blood glucose and may need to modify their menu to help reduce blood sugar spikes. Still, eliminating entire food groups generally isn't necessary when it comes to diabetes. Talk to your doctor for guidance in your specific situation, but in general, people don't have to avoid sugar or carbohydrates entirely in order to manage their blood sugar (despite diet culture's messages to the contrary).

In fact, it's really not helpful to cut out carbs altogether because they are essential for brain function. An inadequate supply of carbs can leave you feeling tired, foggy-headed, and hangry. You might simply need to learn how carbs work in your particular body and how to work with them. Again, that's where attuned eating comes into play.

With diabetes, that might mean tuning into how you feel when you're hungry, full, and in between, and monitoring your blood sugar to see how it relates to those physical sensations. Once you've started to learn your body's signs, you can use them to help you recognize which food combinations and eating times help you feel satisfied and energized, and which ones make you feel low in energy or send your blood sugar out of whack. Including protein and fat in meals and snacks, in addition to carbohydrates, is often helpful for people with diabetes looking to manage blood sugar. If you need support in this process, look for a registered dietitian or certified diabetes care and education specialist who is knowledgeable about intuitive eating and disordered eating recovery.

Another example of a condition that may require some adjustments in eating is high cholesterol. Saturated fat from animal products may contribute to elevated blood cholesterol, which is why many people with this condition are told to reduce their consumption of saturated fat. (Dietary cholesterol, on the other hand, doesn't significantly raise blood cholesterol levels in humans, despite what you may have heard about foods such as eggs in the 1980s and 90s.) Those with high cholesterol might experiment with adding more plant-based proteins and fats to their menu and see if it makes a difference in lab values.

Yet with cholesterol, too, extreme dieting is not generally required—and in fact may be counterproductive, as restriction can increase cholesterol levels. Moreover, if a person's cholesterol is more than a little bit elevated, it often requires the addition of a statin medication and may be impossible to address through dietary changes alone. Indeed, we've seen people go to extremes to avoid saturated fat or pursue weight loss in an effort to treat their high cholesterol, when the only intervention that was successful was medication. Keep in mind that people of all sizes can have elevated cholesterol.

As you can see, although there are some health conditions that may require menu modifications, the need for dietary change is often grossly exaggerated in diet and wellness culture. In addition, there are a number of supposedly "medically necessary" food restrictions that actually aren't—and when you're avoiding foods without a real medical necessity, it can vastly complicate your ability to learn attuned eating and heal from disordered eating.

For example, there's a type of food-intolerance test called IgG testing that some alternative-health providers use on people with digestive disorders. In an IgG test, the lab analyzes your blood for immunoglobulin-G antibodies to food and returns a long list of foods that you're supposedly intolerant to. In fact, the test is not scientifically validated, meaning that it doesn't detect food sensitivities as it claims to do, but instead likely indicates you've been exposed to particular foods and your body is okay with them. (This lack of validity is why IgG tests generally aren't covered by insurance.)

The same is true of many other spurious tests, including hair testing, cell testing, and muscle testing, whose results are no better at predicting food sensitivities than chance. As Christy (Harrison, 2019) wrote in her first book, *Anti-Diet*, "You'd be better off asking a Magic 8 Ball whether you were intolerant to gluten; at least the 8 Ball wouldn't charge you hundreds of dollars out of pocket" (p. 64).

If you've gotten one of those tests and started to feel like you actually do have reactions to the foods it told you to avoid, then it's worth exploring whether you might be experiencing the nocebo effect. This doesn't mean that "it's all in your head"—in fact, quite the opposite. Both the nocebo and placebo effects are testaments to the power of the mind-body connection and to the fact that your beliefs about food can actually cause physical responses. Our intention here isn't to discourage you from listening to your body, but to encourage you to do due diligence around claims that are not verified.

Take a moment to reflect on how you feel after reading this. Are there any diagnoses or dietary restrictions you might reconsider? Are you feeling resistant to that possibility?

_____

_____

_____

_____

_____

_____

One final caveat here: Figuring out how certain foods make you feel is actually a very advanced move because it's hard to disentangle what's coming from diet culture and what's actually coming from how the foods are sitting with you. Early in the intuitive eating process (not to mention in the process of eating disorder recovery), it's hard not to conflate avoiding foods because of how they make you feel with avoiding them because you've labeled them as bad. The mind-body connection is so powerful that guilt about eating a particular food can actually cause physical pain.

If you suspect that's going on for you, and if you have reliable access to food, you might try experimenting with giving yourself full, unconditional permission to eat the foods that diet and wellness culture have told you are bad. Try to do this without judgment and observe how you feel.

_____

_____

_____

_____

If any symptoms come up, you can investigate the role that your anxiety about the food might be playing—is it making you hyper-scrutinize your digestion for any sign of discomfort? Are you experiencing that classic pit-of-the-stomach manifestation of anxiety that's making it hard to eat? Write about your experiences here.

_____

_____

_____

_____

It can be a delicate balance between listening to your body and making sure the diet culture voice in your head isn't creating symptoms that wouldn't otherwise be there. Give yourself as much time, space, and support as possible to figure it all out.

Media Literacy

Media outlets love to report on new studies in health, wellness, and nutrition—in large part because those kinds of stories get clicked, shared, and spread around widely, resulting in more subscribers, ad dollars, and clout for the publication (and in some cases the reporter).

Unfortunately, media reporting on such studies leaves a lot to be desired. This is especially true when it comes to studies showing apparent links between certain kinds of food and health outcomes. Even if the research only shows a correlation—which, as we've discussed, is not the same thing as causation—headlines and articles still often frame it in causal terms: "Eating chocolate may lower risk of X" or "Red meat could be increasing your risk of Y."

This framing is problematic because it typically leaves out discussion of other important factors that could be responsible for the apparent link, such as demographic or behavioral differences in the groups of people who tend to eat more or less of a certain food. These differences are called *confounding factors*, and they're all too common in nutrition research.

Every time a new study comes out that supposedly shows the risks or benefits of eating a certain way, keep in mind that there are likely some major confounding factors at play in these studies that almost never get controlled for.

One of those is disordered eating. When researchers ask people questions about what they typically eat, they don't generally ask *how* they eat—whether they're dieting, restricting, bingeing, compensating, or using any other disordered behaviors. When those researchers then draw conclusions about health based on people's self-reported habits (e.g., "People with higher sugar consumption have higher levels of XYZ disease"), they don't account for the fact that *disordered behaviors with food* might be a driver of those health outcomes, rather than the food itself.

The same is true for weight science. Of all the studies claiming that higher weights are "unhealthy," we've never seen any that controlled for weight stigma or weight cycling as confounding factors—when in fact, weight stigma and weight cycling can account for many, if not all, of the negative health outcomes experienced by people in larger bodies. So, when you see fear-inducing headlines about new nutrition or weight studies, try to remember it's extremely unlikely that the study tells the whole story (or that the news report is even telling the whole story about the study, for that matter).

The next time you see a media report about nutrition, take a moment to reflect on how it's making you feel. What emotions or physical sensations are coming up for you?

_____

_____

_____

_____

Now imagine that you were to rewrite the piece from a critical lens, given all that you've learned in this workbook. What inaccuracies would you want to correct in the piece (e.g., the assumption that correlation equals causation, the failure to account for social determinants of health)? How would you frame the information to help reduce fear and shame in your audience?

_____

_____

_____

_____

_____

_____

SIFT Through Misinformation

When you come across wellness information online, you might try using a method called SIFT, which was developed by a media literacy researcher at the University of Washington named Mike Caulfield (2023). SIFT stands for its four steps:

1. **S**top.

2. **I**nvestigate the source.

3. **F**ind better coverage.

4. **T**race claims, quotes, and media to the original context.

When it comes to information about diet and wellness culture, **stop** means that you pause before you decide to overhaul your diet, buy a "wellness plan" or weight loss program, share the message on social media, subscribe to a mailing list, and so on. Take a moment to calm your nervous system before you react. This not only saves you from wasting your money or getting pulled back into disordered eating, but it also can help keep you from inadvertently spreading misinformation. Think of it as a temporary information quarantine.

Next, **investigating the source** means looking into whether the information is coming from a reputable channel. In the wellness context, this generally means a well-conducted scientific study or a provider with recognized credentials, who isn't taking money from the diet or diet-drug industries. Ask questions like: Are this source's claims about food and weight aligned with the principles of recovery from disordered eating and diet culture? Or are they encouraging you to cut out entire food groups (like carbs, fat, gluten, or dairy), skip meals, restrict your eating to certain windows, label foods as good and bad, take drugs to shrink your body, or engage in other practices that are likely to put your healing at risk?

Find better coverage is about looking to reputable sources of health and wellness information that you've come to trust over time, like your medical doctor, your psychotherapist, your dietitian, certain publications, and so forth. If these sources are skeptical of the claims, that's important to consider. It's also helpful to consider whether reputable publications are *not* covering a claim that seems impressive (e.g., that following a certain diet or wellness plan can cure cancer or reverse disease). Remember that traditional media outlets are always looking for the "next big thing" in nutrition, but they also have a mandate to fact-check their coverage (unlike influencers and unlicensed wellness practitioners). So if they're not reporting on something that's a big story among wellness influencers, that might be a red flag that there's no solid evidence behind it.

Finally, **tracing claims, quotes, and media to the original context** means that you don't just take the word of a social media post or headline, but actually track down where the claim originated and learn the full story. You don't necessarily have to wade into full scientific studies—while that can certainly be helpful, most people don't have training in how to parse scientific research or even have access to the full studies, since many are behind steep paywalls. But you can usually get a decent sense of the findings from the abstract (a free summary of the study), especially the results section. If you look at that section and see terms like *association*, *link*, or *correlation* (or cautious language such as *may be linked to* or *may increase the risk*), then the study isn't able to say anything about causation.

And if there *isn't* a study that supports the claims, that's clearly another red flag. Unfortunately, some wellness influencers, including some well-known medical doctors, have been known to "cite" studies that don't actually have anything to do with the claim they're making, perhaps figuring that very few people will ever bother to click the link and read the study. And certainly many of us don't have time for that in our busy lives! But if you're seriously considering believing a health or wellness claim, it's worth taking your time to really check it out. When you do, you may be surprised to find that there's no real evidence to support it, even if the footnotes make it look otherwise.

Take a moment to think of a nutrition or wellness claim that has hooked you but that you suspect may be false. Apply the SIFT method to the claim and note your experience:

1. Stop. How does it feel when you do this?

_____

_____

_____

_____

2. Investigate the source. What do you find about them?

_____

_____

_____

_____

3. Find better coverage. What coverage do you find, and what does it say?

_____

_____

_____

_____

4. Trace claims, quotes, and media to the original context. Can you find the original context? And if so, does it support the claim? Or is the truth more complicated?

_____

_____

_____

_____

The reality is that if we live long enough, virtually everyone will develop health conditions over time. Eating or avoiding certain foods can't prevent that. No single food or food group will make you live forever. Anything that makes those kinds of promises is, sadly, just too good to be true.

And so we've come full circle: Eating a wide variety of foods based on your preferences is most likely the best option to support your physical and emotional well-being.

Clinician's Corner

Throughout your career, you will inevitably see clients with health conditions and concerns. For many clients, one of your most important roles as a clinician will be to help them navigate these issues without spiraling into disordered eating.

Unfortunately, it can be a slippery slope from receiving a health diagnosis to making drastic dietary changes and becoming extremely fearful of food. Even in cases where some menu modifications are supported by solid science, some clients may hear (and some health care providers may communicate) a message that's far more restrictive than the evidence warrants. This advice is especially dangerous if restriction for the purpose of weight loss is recommended. It's also concerning if the client's diagnosis was inaccurate (e.g., a "food sensitivity" diagnosis made on the basis of an IgG test or another problematic testing method) because in those cases, there's no genuine reason to avoid foods—and many potential downsides.

No clinician can be expected to know the science (or lack thereof) behind every diagnosis, especially in disciplines that aren't their own. But we'd encourage you *not* to simply support clients' dietary restrictions without first exploring them in depth, both with the client and, if possible, with their other health care providers. If a client's food restrictions are causing them distress or contributing to a disordered mindset about food, it may be worth encouraging the client to get a second opinion from a health professional (ideally one who is well versed in disordered eating, though we recognize that may not always be possible), as well as perhaps investigating the scientific evidence for any dietary modifications yourself.

Keep in mind that even in conditions where dietary restrictions are seen as a given, such as diabetes, usually there is still plenty of room for flexibility. Having a medical condition may make it more challenging for your clients to develop a peaceful relationship with food, but it doesn't make it impossible; it may just require additional support in untangling the layers of food fears. In general, we find that if clients have ended the deprivation that comes from the diet mindset, they're in a much stronger position to make any adjustments in their food intake for the purpose of supporting their bodies from a place of self-care.

It is also important to acknowledge that not only can health diagnoses put people at risk of disordered eating, but in some cases, they may lead clients to pursue unproven and potentially harmful treatments. This may happen when clients see alternative-health or integrative-health providers who recommend such treatments, as well as when clients search online for help for their conditions and get exposed to misinformation. People who are suffering from painful or difficult symptoms and who feel dismissed by the health care system may be especially susceptible to risky treatments because they are feeling desperate. For clients who do find themselves on that slippery slope while working with you, it can be helpful to stay focused on how their dietary restrictions and other interventions are affecting them and their relationships with food and their bodies.

If you are a therapist and have clients with health conditions such as high cholesterol or diabetes, we recommend collaborating with an intuitive eating dietitian who can ensure that any health-related menu modifications are evidence-based and truly necessary for the client's specific situation. The key is for clients to make any needed dietary changes that are in service of supporting the body rather than for the purpose of weight loss. It's helpful to have clients consider that "making the match" can not only be about what tastes good and offers satisfaction, but also what supports their bodies' needs.

And for dietitians, it can be helpful to refer clients to a psychotherapist who can support them in the deeper work of dealing with health concerns. With a strong support system, clients will be better able to navigate the sometimes rough waters of managing chronic conditions in diet and wellness culture.

CHAPTER 9

Challenging Diet Culture

Throughout this workbook, you've become aware that the diet mindset keeps you stuck in a cycle that creates physical and emotional harm. You've learned ways to heal your relationship with food as you eat for nourishment and pleasure. You've come to understand that if you've experienced trauma, food may have become a coping mechanism that allowed you to survive. You've considered the idea that bodies come in all shapes and sizes and that there are strategies to reject internalized weight stigma. You've discovered new ways to think about health and take care of your body to support your physical and emotional well-being, whether or not you lose weight as a side effect. You've gathered information to help you evaluate claims around food and wellness. It's been a long journey!

But the work doesn't end with our workbook. Given the power of diet and wellness culture, no matter where you're at in your own process, you will encounter shaming messages about food and weight. You will also encounter claims that weight loss is both possible and necessary.

At the same time, there are a growing number of clinicians, health professionals, and laypeople rejecting the weight loss framework and coming to the same conclusions we've talked about throughout this workbook. As you embrace an anti-diet approach, you become part of that change. Whether it's in your personal or professional life, challenging diet culture is something we can all be part of so that future generations can feel more at home in their bodies and at peace with food.

Imagine that you woke up one morning and discovered that your body, as it is right now, is accepted by the world around you. Your family, friends, and colleagues embrace you just as you are. Your health care professionals no longer focus on body shape or size. Your body type—as well as your skin color, gender identity, age, and ability—is represented in mainstream magazines, TV, film, and commercials.

Use this space to describe how that would make you feel and what would be different in your life.

_____

_____

_____

_____

_____

_____

Changing diet culture takes place as people take actions to challenge it, and you can be part of that change. In this chapter, we'll explore ways to reject diet culture messages that you continue to receive and consider ways to make sure you're not reinforcing the culture. You don't have to do this alone. There are many other people who are making the same decision to let go of a diet mindset and embrace the idea that people of all shapes and sizes deserve to feel at home in their bodies and be treated with respect.

Speaking Up

As you let go of the diet mindset and move toward greater body acceptance, it's important to decide how you'll share (or not share) your journey. It may be protective for you *not* to explain what you're doing because you're not certain enough yet of how to describe this approach, or it's too exhausting to defend yourself. Or perhaps there is someone in your life who has already concluded that diets don't work and is on a similar path, so sharing your experiences feels supportive.

No matter what, there will likely be times when you encounter diet culture and need to decide how to respond. Here are some suggestions for managing diet conversations, navigating weight loss compliments, speaking out against diet culture, building resilience, and finding community.

Managing Diet Conversations

Remember that in letting go of the diet mindset and moving toward attuned eating, you've been learning a new language when it comes to food and weight. However, this is a new language that important people in your life may not be able to understand. Here are some reasons they may not be able to support you at this point in time:

- They have internalized cultural messages about dieting, weight, and health. Mainstream thinking still promotes the thinner body as the healthier body and views dieting as the way to achieve the "ideal" weight. These messages become entrenched, and it takes active unlearning to shift these views. While you've been doing this unlearning via this workbook and other resources, they're still caught in the diet culture mindset.

- They are stuck in their own body negativity. Since body dissatisfaction is the norm in our culture, it's often hard for people to imagine that there is a different way to view their bodies. Your decision to end the diet cycle, and the reasons behind that decision, feel threatening to them because they aren't yet ready to let go of the belief that they can attain thinness and all of the promises of happiness, attractiveness, health, and success that are supposed to come with weight loss. To do so feels like giving up to them.

- They benefit from your body shame or are invested in your thinness. For example, parents or caregivers sometimes feel that their child's body size is a reflection of their parenting skills. They may experience shame about their own body size and believe that helping their child become or stay thinner will allow them to have a better life. Unfortunately, despite what may seem like good intentions, this lack of acceptance can lead a child to feel devalued or worthless, and these feelings often continue into adulthood.

Because diet conversations are normative in our culture, it likely that you will hear comments about dieting, food, and weight from friends, family, coworkers, and others. Setting boundaries is key when it comes to diet talk. You have the right to decide what foods satisfy you and how you savor your food. You also have the right to say, "No, thank you" when you don't want to eat something.

Take a moment and think about what you have experienced when people around you bring up the topic of dieting.

_____

_____

_____

_____

_____

To begin setting boundaries around diet conversations, visualize a situation you've been in where someone started a conversation based on the diet mindset, commented on what you were eating, or used body-shaming language. Consider which of the following responses you might use in the future. We've left extra space for you to come up with your own responses. Always remember that you deserve to hold on to your own truth.

- "Instead of talking about diets, I'd love to hear about your new relationship [or otherwise change the subject]."
- "I respect that each of us gets to decide what's best for our bodies. I hope you can respect that talking about diets isn't helpful to me, so I'd like to keep that out of our conversations."
- "I know you want what's best for me. I've decided that dieting isn't good for my health, but I'm finding other ways to support my body. I hope you understand, but either way, I am asking you not to talk about weight with me."
- "I appreciate your perspective, but I've found for myself that diet talk is counterproductive."
- "I know what's best for my body. Let's talk about something else."
- "I know that everyone talks about dieting, but I've come to learn why it's not a good idea. I'd be glad to share more, if you like."
- Additional ideas: _____

_____

_____

_____

It's also important to think about what other kinds of conversations nourish you. What do you want to share about yourself? What do you want to know about others? Finding authentic ways to connect around life experiences, interests, challenges, and dreams leads to more satisfying and connected relationships. Use this space to reflect on what kinds of conversations nourish you.

_____

_____

_____

_____

_____

Navigating Weight Loss Compliments

As you stop dieting, there's no way to know where your body will land. You may gain weight, lose weight, or stay the same. (Remember that if you lose weight, it's a side effect of the work you're doing to make peace with food, not the goal or a sign of success.)

We've also had clients who've been told they look great because they've "lost weight" when they don't believe that their body size has actually changed. They're feeling better because they're no longer at war with their bodies, and it seems that in diet culture, when someone feels better, it is assumed that they've lost weight.

Part of shifting diet culture is ending the act of commenting on other people's bodies. At the same time, when someone loses weight, there's a good chance they want you to notice that they're thinner. After all, they've worked hard and deprived themselves to get there! So what should you do when they're pointing out their change in body size and clearly want you to say something?

Our clients have responded by finding phrases that acknowledge the person's request without being complicit in the cycle of shame. Examples include:

- "I'm glad you're feeling good. I wish you all the best."
- "I cared about you before, and I care about you now. Your body size doesn't change that."

Add your own ideas for responses here. The more you can visualize ways to respond, the better prepared you'll be if and when the time comes.

_____

_____

_____

_____

_____

On the flip side, if you're on the receiving end of weight loss compliments, think about how to respond. Saying thank you typically feels like you're participating in diet culture, so it's helpful to imagine what else you could say if someone gives you a weight loss compliment. Here are some examples:

- "I don't really keep track of my weight anymore. But I am feeling good."
- "I know you mean well, but I think that commenting on bodies isn't good for anyone."

Add your own ideas for responses here. Again, the more you can visualize responding in these ways, the better prepared you'll be if and when the time comes.

_____

_____

_____

_____

_____

Finally, we want to acknowledge that we all like to get compliments! Consider the people who are important to you and think about what you might compliment them on other than body size or shape. Do they have a good sense of humor? Are they wearing fun earrings? Are they passionate about a hobby? Have they been an important support for you lately? There are so many ways to let people know what you enjoy or appreciate about them without commenting on their body.

What qualities could you compliment people on that aren't related to their body size?

_____

_____

_____

_____

What would you like people to notice about *you* that's not related to your body size?

_____

_____

_____

_____

_____

Taking Anti-Diet Action

One of our workshop participants recently commented, "Once you know about the harm of diet culture, you can't unknow it," and this is the experience of most people who let go of the diet mindset. With this new mentality, you'll likely notice that you're more sensitive to messages everywhere that value thinness over the natural diversity of body size and that promote the pursuit of weight loss. When you encounter these stigmatizing messages, you can decide if and how you want to use your voice to reject them.

Think about whether there are any actions you want to take at this time to help challenge diet culture. These may involve personal rejections of diet culture or actions that you take in a more public forum. How you feel about taking action can change over time, so be sure to reflect on this activity on a regular basis. We'll give you some examples, and you can add more based on your own needs and energy level:

- Write a blog post about your own experiences with making peace with food or rejecting diet culture.

- Wear clothes that are comfortable for your body.

- Create a book club for anti-diet and body acceptance books (or this workbook!).

- Eat dessert without apology.

- Write a letter to the editor in response to news articles that show anti-fat bias.

- Speak out about policies that promote weight stigma, such as routine weigh-ins at medical appointments, BMI report cards in the school system, or work policies that give financial discounts to employees based on weight in the name of wellness.

- Add your own ideas here: _____

  _____

  _____

  _____

Remember, you are the pebble that will create the ripples to help change diet culture.

Building Resilience

Even as you become more grounded in the anti-diet approach, you may find yourself struggling when others aren't able to understand your journey. One strategy to help you build resilience through these times is known as the 3 R's (Harrison & Matz, 2021):

- **Remind** yourself that your weight is the result of complex factors (including genetics, yo-yo dieting, medications, health conditions, and more).

- **Reject** weight stigma rather than internalizing it.

- **Repeat**, "I deserve to be treated with respect at any size."